Medicinema – Doctors in Films

Medicinema – Doctors in Films

BRIAN GLASSER

Teaching Fellow, Medical Humanities
University College London Medical School

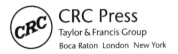

CRC Press

Taylor & Francis Group

Boca Raton London New York

CRC Press is an imprint of the
Taylor & Francis Group, an **informa** business

Radcliffe Publishing Ltd
33–41 Dallington Street
London
EC1V 0BB
United Kingdom

www.radcliffe-oxford.com

Electronic catalogue and worldwide online ordering facility.

British Library Cataloguing in Publication Data

A catalogue record for this book is available from the British Library.

ISBN-13: 978 184619 157 2

The paper used for the text pages of this book is FSC® certified. FSC (The Forest Stewardship Council®) is an international network to promote responsible management of the world's forests.

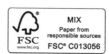

Typeset by Pindar NZ, Auckland, New Zealand

Contents

Acknowledgements

I am very grateful to Pauline Bryant, Michael Clark, Trish Greenhalgh, Joe Rosenthal and Graham Woodroffe for supplying important nutrients en route. I also thank John Salinsky – for his chapter, naturally; but also for his implacable commitment to medical education of the broadest and deepest kind, a model for us all. Then there are the students who have bravely and curiously signed up for my courses over the last ten-plus years, and contributed to the explorations thereon that have led to this book (in particular, those who took the late lamented BSc in medical humanities that ran between 2003 and 2006 at what used to be called the Royal Free and University College Medical School). Among these, Lydia Collingridge, Rory Conn and Nick Hulme were especially helpful, undertaking invaluable background work for Chapter 6.

The term 'Medicinema' came to me over ten years ago and I started to use it as a title for lectures and courses. I subsequently discovered a charity with this name that organises film screenings for patients in healthcare settings (www.medicinema.org.uk) – a wonderful enterprise. I think this town is big enough for both of us.

This book is dedicated to Chips Glasser,
who would have enjoyed it; and to Jeanette,
who I think will.

'J'aime les films qui me font rêver, mais je n'aime
pas qu'on rêve à ma place.'
('I like films that make me dream, but I don't like
[film-makers] dreaming on my behalf.')

Georges Franju (1912–87)

CHAPTER 1

Introduction: medicine through a lens

The title of this book is a manifesto, its elision being less straightforward than it may at first appear – 'cinema' is derived from the Greek *kinema*, meaning 'movement'; while 'medicine' comes from the Latin *medicere*, to heal. So the Greeks and Romans – two hefty civilisations – here dovetail nicely; as I hope (*pace* CP Snow) will Art and Science in the pages that follow.

Nor let us typecast. Medicine, notwithstanding its evidence bases and algorithms, is an artistic science, as people have become increasingly aware; and film has always been one of the more scientific arts. The development of 'movies' in the 1890s from still photography (itself a nineteenth-century invention) was due to the efforts of scientists who envisaged putting the new medium to their own use. And subsequently it could be argued that the history of cinema has been written by scientific advances: its progressions from silent cinema to talkies, from black-and-white to colour to cinemascope to digital; through the development of film stock, lenses, lightweight cameras, computer-generated images, and so on. Thus the aesthetics have always been driven, at least in part, by technology. In view of all this, cross-cultural studies would seem to be fertile ground; and this book represents a new log thrown on the fire that has been burning steadily for some years (see the work of Shortland (1989), Jouhanneau (1994), Dans (2000), Flores (2004), Friedman (2004), and Harper and Moor (2005), to name just a few).

Moreover, film and medicine have been linked since the earliest days of cinema. Film historians tell us that medicine was the first profession to be depicted in fictional films (Shortland, 1989) – before even cowboys, criminals or the clergy. And since then it is astonishing how many big stars have acted as doctors – from major silent thespians such as John Barrymore, through 1930s matinee idols such as Ronald Coleman and Clark Gable, to modern-day equivalents such as Tom Cruise or Keanu Reeves (with a few in between that stretch credibility beyond breaking point, such as Frank Sinatra and Elvis Presley). This is a clear indicator of the more or less continuous commercial potential of medical films (big names cost money, which needs to be recouped) – that is, the public like them.

Furthermore, we are not dealing with regular but rare star vehicles alone. It is nigh on impossible to accurately list the number of films in which a doctor has had a substantial role – notwithstanding the heroic efforts of some of the writers referred to earlier, along with Paietta and Kauppila (1999) – let alone those in which medics feature in bit parts or cameos.

How can this prevalence be explained? One factor certainly is the universality of sickness and, by extension – at least for most modern viewers in the developed world– of doctors and medicine. Some of us may have had dealings with lawyers; but all of us have surely visited a doctor. (On top of which, the issue under discussion with them, namely our health, is probably more important to us than legal matters, at least in broad terms.) In theory, this might lead to a huge quantity of 'sickness' films; and indeed there are a considerable number of these (Glasser, 2005). However, sickness – and again this is a generalisation – might be perceived by audiences (and film-makers) to have a relatively narrow emotional range; and a fairly gruelling one at that. By concentrating on the doctors, we are allowed to experience a cleaner contact with disease, at one remove – doctors are intimately involved with it, but do not 'have' it; and they can walk away from the sickbed and its (possible) attendant physical and emotional mess. Moreover, with a bit of luck they will be responsible for a heroic cure or two, and as mentioned above, the saviour is often more attractive than the saved (note the active and passive roles implicit in that phrase!). Similarly, medical films are one way in which the movie industry can cater for people who enjoy life-or-death dramas that do not involve guns and ticking time bombs.

In this relatively secular age, a GP will probably know more about the local community than the parish priest, rabbi or vicar. Doctors are given privileged access to private matters in the real world, affording the cinema audience a chance to be vicariously nosy in the reel world. Of course, films (and not just medical ones) are intrinsically voyeuristic – we go to see them at least in part because we enjoy watching other people's lives in varying states of intimacy. And perhaps there is a spectator sport element in medical practice, too.

Certainly a healthy curiosity about others would seem to be a *sine qua non* for entering the medical profession.

Then there is the versatility of doctors. They can be of any adult age, either gender, any class (at least on entry to medical school), and from pretty much any place or era; and perform any number of functions, from pronouncing a body dead to keeping one alive in desperate circumstances. This allows doctors (and through them medicine) to be deployed plausibly in an almost limitless number of ways.

If one accepts, then, the phenomenon of medicinema, what do we make of it? For the utilitarian, there are several ready answers to this question; and they have been well represented in another compound-noun-titled book, *Cinemeducation* (Alexander *et al.*, 2005), which lays out many of the headings that medical students will find in their curriculum (geriatric medicine, eating disorders, sexual dysfunction, and so on) and links them to clips from films that can be used as teaching aids. The approach is nicely complementary to that adopted in this book. Rather than starting with medicine and moving on to film, I do the reverse. I am interested in what films have to say about doctors and doctoring – in how medicine looks through a lens. Therefore in this book you will find a chapter on a great director, rather than an epidemic; or on a single entire film rather than a collection of clips.[1] The sociologist in me is wary of medicalisation – that is, the belief, often ingrained and therefore unrecognised, that all life comes under one ICD heading or another. Yet, although film is not a handmaiden to medicine, it can teach us to look, listen, analyse and interpret – all fundamental skills in most medical practice.

This book attempts to draw a relatively small number of the many films that feature doctors into groupings around some fairly heterogeneous themes. The groupings could quite easily have been otherwise (the same hand of cards can be organised according to suits, numbers, and so on), which is of course not to say that they are arbitrary. The aim is to give the reader some stimulating starting points for watching the chosen films and others beyond.

This hardly needs to be stated, but I have not seen every film that includes

---

1 Of course clips will be discussed too, and I don't want to overstate the bipolarity of the two books, for there are naturally points of overlap. Indeed, there are other approaches. For example, John Salinsky, who has contributed a chapter to this book, regularly shows his GP trainees films that (horror of horrors) don't have any doctors or patients in them at all. He does so in the belief that being exposed to great art is *ipso facto* beneficial to doctors (and to the rest of us, too).

a doctor in its cast of characters. So there are certainly movies out there that do not fall within the schemas I have created in my chapters. And, strange though it may seem, film-makers have not always conformed to those schemas. Therefore this book does not attempt to be comprehensive; rather, it is a miscellany, designed to draw out what I hope are some interesting themes. Indeed, to my thinking, incompleteness is a virtue because it prompts the reader to venture forth on their own journeys of discovery. With that in mind, I have tried to talk enough about the films to give a flavour of their attractions without in the process pre-empting (what I trust will be) the reader's desire to see them.

My selection process has been unapologetically subjective. There were some obvious choices: films with titles such as *The Doctor* or *The Hospital* surely had to be discussed. But what about *Windom's Way* or *Le Corbeau* (even when it is translated as *The Raven*)? I hope to draw attention to films with great merits, such as these two, that might otherwise fly under the radar. Similarly, there may be a slight bias towards older films in the book, because they are less well known these days, and so require more publicity if they are not to be forgotten. Plenty of old films are best left in the past, but not the ones in this book.

(Nor has this presented difficulties on a practical level. Happily, the trend is towards ever greater availability of films. VHS tape came first of course, enabling people to easily watch and re-watch movies they might have waited a while to catch on television or in the cinema. The informed reissuing of back catalogues has grown apace since the advent of DVD, and no doubt in the future it will eventually be possible to summon everything at home down a wire. At the time of writing, only a tiny percentage of the films discussed in this book cannot be obtained using a computer, the Internet and a little effort. It should be emphasised that this domestic consumption is *faute de mieux*. Films are meant to be seen in cinemas – they pack more punch there, and the visceral side of the art should never be underestimated. However, in this other sector of the ecosystem the situation is less cheery, and it is now much more difficult to see non-contemporary films in theatrical screenings than in days of yore.)

Doubtless I have adopted this approach for egocentric reasons. I am a non-medic with an arts and social science background who has been teaching in medical schools and on postgraduate courses for 20 years (I would call myself a fifth-columnist, except that I have been undisguised throughout), and I have a deep-seated belief in the benefit of out-of-body (of knowledge) experiences, especially in this instance, in a field that offers a refracted image of medicine.

One of the first steps is to accord proper respect to this other field. Film studies is a well-established international academic discipline. To understand an art form better, it behoves us to learn about it. There is an intrinsic asymmetry between the many people and many hours (in fact the many days, months and years) that it takes to make a film and one person seeing it in 100 consecutive minutes. Therefore it is almost inevitable that the spectator will not 'get' everything in one viewing (this is notwithstanding the various subterfuges that cinema uses to go about its business). Like most things, practice is important. The more films you watch, and the more actively you watch them, the better the return on your time will be when you see one. To watch a film actively, you need to do the sorts of things that are covered within film studies courses; and I hope that this book will, *en passant*, be of assistance with regard to this.

Thus forewarned and forearmed, you are invited to give your ticket to the usher and take your seat as the lights go down . . .

References

Alexander M, Lenahan P, Pavlov A. *Cinemeducation: a comprehensive guide to using film in medical education.* Oxford: Radcliffe Publishing; 2005.

Dans P. *Doctors in the Movies.* Bloomington, IL: Medi-Ed Press; 2000.

Flores G. Doctors in the movies: healers, heels, and Hollywood. *Arch Dis Child.* 2004; 89: 1084–8.

Friedman LD (ed.) *Cultural Sutures: medicine and media.* Durham, NC: Duke University Press; 2004.

Glasser B. Magic bullets, dark victories and cold comforts: some preliminary observations about stories of sickness in the cinema. In: Harper G, Moor A (eds) *Signs of Life: medicine and cinema.* London: Wallflower Press; 2005.

Harper G, Moor A (eds) *Signs of Life: medicine and cinema.* London: Wallflower Press; 2005.

Jouhanneau J. Les scientifiques vus par les cineastes. In: Martinet A (ed.) *Le Cinéma et la Science.* Paris: CNRS Éditions; 1994. pp. 248–61.

Paietta A, Kauppila J. *Health Professionals on Screen.* London: Scarecrow Press; 1999.

Shortland M. *Medicine and Film: a checklist, survey and research resource.* Oxford: Wellcome Unit for the History of Medicine; 1989.

CHAPTER 2

Beware Greeks bearing gifts, especially one called Hippocrates

It might seem odd that a profession that supposedly exists to bring solace to humanity should be so closely associated with the horror genre in the cinema. However, a little reflection ought to banish such naivety, because medicine can certainly be frightening, and fears projected large are the stuff of horror. Think of swallowing a substance that will change you, perhaps irreversibly, and in ways over which you have little or no control. Think of being injected with something that will put you to sleep, and on waking finding that your body is altered (visibly or invisibly). Doctors may become accustomed to such phenomena because of their daily dealings with them, and patients with chronic or life-threatening conditions may come to terms with them, too; but for most people most of the time these possibilities induce a degree of anxiety.

Such fears are essentially somatic – they are about what might be done to our bodies. However, there is a psychological aspect at play here, too, which relates to process rather than outcome. It is much more frightening when a person who comes under the cover of beneficence proves to have bad intentions – that is, when someone who is kind turns out to be cruel. We know where we stand with conventional villains (in films, as in life). They are on the opposing side, and we can be afraid of them straightforwardly. However, doctors start off, by definition, on our side. Their job is completely and unambiguously concerned with helping us; and accordingly we trust them. What, then, if that trust is breached? What if we, willingly but unknowingly, are putting our life in the hands of someone who wants to terminate it? That way lies real horror; and it is impossible not to end this paragraph with a name: Harold Shipman.

Horror film history

Horror movies are the hardy perennials of the cinema garden. This fact has caused commentators to realise belatedly that their popularity might be because of, rather than despite, the semi-detached relationship of these films with reality. Starting from that insight, the horror genre becomes a particularly interesting expression of the human psyche; and a rich seam for psychoanalytic film theorists, who point to all manner of repressed issues and regressive behaviour being manifested in these films. (Perhaps exaggeration is the natural rhetoric for expressing repressed anxieties.) In simple terms, we can see how horror movies allow us to explore some of our most fundamental fears in a safe way. No matter how weird and terrifying the film may be, it ends, and we then return to the contained normality of the real world. (This is true of other types of film, too, of course, but the horror label allows a degree of exaggeration and fantasy that would be difficult to accommodate in dramas in the realist tradition.)

Horror films had their most celebrated flowering in the early 1930s in America. Think of classics such as *The Invisible Man*, *The Mummy* and *Dracula*, as well as perhaps the most durable duo of the lot – *Frankenstein* and *Dr Jekyll and Mr Hyde*. You may not have seen these films, but the chances are that you will have heard of them, and could sketch out their storylines. (Note, too, that most of them have doctors at their centre, and all include medics somewhere.) All of these oft-revisited stories were filmed in their most famous versions between 1930 and 1933, and provided templates for much of what has followed in the genre. The dates are not arbitrary. This was a very specific moment in American film history. The advent of sound at the end of the 1920s had opened up a new range of (mainly dialogue-related) possibilities that helped to modernise film's surface content; and the Production Code (the so-called Hay's Office Code) of 1930 – which did the opposite, closing off a whole range of content options – had not yet been stringently enforced. Under the Code's aegis, American films from 1933 until the 1960s were to be systematically sanitised, forced into a straitjacket from which only the most subtle and talented filmic Houdinis escaped. Openness about sex, sacrilege, successful wrongdoing – indeed anything that might quicken the breathing of a member of the League of Decency – was suppressed, in a giant exercise in denial. The hope, as with all censorship, was that what you couldn't see wasn't there. However, in this early 1930s halcyon period (from an artistic point of view) the forces of free expression were pushing hard at the limits of acceptability; and horror, with doctors in the vanguard, was one of the crack squadrons.

In *Murders in the Rue Morgue* (Florey, 1932), Dr Mirakle (Bela Lugosi, bringing his Dracula accent with him) abducts young women so that he can experiment with bridging the evolutionary gap between apes and man. His day job (although it takes place at night) involves working as the presenter of a carnival sideshow in Paris that features Erik the Ape Man, an intelligent primate with whom he conducts conversations on stage (albeit in Ape rather than English). Further into the night, however, Mirakle pursues his real interest of trying to crossbreed Erik with a human so as to prove his theory of evolution.[2] His proposed method, although it is never clearly elaborated, involves transfusing blood; but there are several indications that Erik would like to pursue more conventional ways of mixing bodily fluids (insofar as an ape having sexual intercourse with a woman is conventional).[3]

It would take a brave person to argue that the half-cocked way in which the story is played out, and the near-imbecilic characterisation of several of the protagonists, do not compromise a contemporary viewer's enjoyment of this movie (it manages to be too long at a running time of 59 minutes!). Nevertheless, the film offers many pleasures, and even some horror; and they mostly stem from the great cameraman Karl Freund. His exceptional ability to paint with light allows him to create powerful images of menace and beauty – notably when Mirakle is stalking the heroine or experimenting on a hapless female; and the elegant, perceptive mobility of his camera is a joy. These elements ensure that while the dialogue is often stilted (although Mirakle does

---

2   The film is set in 1845, so he was some years ahead of Darwin on this. It is a common device in medical horror movies to blur the distinction between the hero and the villain in the early stages of the film. Thus Mirakle is more 'correct' by our lights (notwithstanding the recent resurgence of creationism) than the audiences at his sideshow who mock his theories and call him a heretic. Also, Dupin (the hero of the tale) is a medical student who himself acquires bodies for study by illicit means (by bribing the city official in charge of the morgue). His flatmate even notes that the glassy-eyed stare he is developing as a result of sleepless nights devoted to research makes him look a little like Mirakle.

3   Erik – 'the beast with a human soul' – clearly prefigures King Kong, who hit the screen only a year later. The rooftop climax of *Murders in the Rue Morgue* was also echoed, somewhat upgraded, in the later film.

have some good lines), the visual experience is so atmospheric that the film amply repays the watching.

There is an overlap of theme between this film and the poetically titled *Island of Lost Souls* (Kenton, 1932), which is set in the (then) present day. On an uncharted island somewhere in the South Seas, Dr Moreau is attempting to hasten the evolution of animals into humans. This is a more substantial film than *Murders in the Rue Morgue*, and offers an early version of an ethical theme that runs through the history of medical horror (and many non-horror medical films, too) – that of whether the ends can justify the means. Moreau continues to employ research methods that had seen him run out of London 'with angry England at my heels.' He is assisted by a doctor who he scooped up during departure who 'was facing a prison term for a professional indiscretion.' Inside his compound, Moreau undertakes vivisection without qualms in a room that the island dwellers (a hideous bunch of his failed prototypes) call the House of Pain. We may initially harbour some sympathy for Mirakle, but Moreau is so single-minded that the audience never doubts that he is a wrong-doer.[4] When challenged about the agonies that he inflicts on dumb creatures, he replies 'What does that matter?' It is an unapologetic attitude that, allied to scenes featuring figures screaming on the operating table, was sufficiently shocking for the film to be banned for 27 years in England (although this may say more about the fondness of the English for animals than anything else). Notwithstanding his barbarity, Moreau is a wonderful creation thanks to the distinguished English actor who plays him, Charles Laughton. Against horror convention, he unsettles us not by ranting and raving, but by speaking extraordinarily quietly and with the decorum of an English colonial gentleman, a sly smile never far from his lips. He sprinkles irony lightly on a number of his utterances, giving the film a macabre modernity that belies its age.

Sources and successors

Although the early 1930s gave birth to the so-called Golden Age of Horror (a lovely oxymoron), this was no immaculate conception. There were important cinematic antecedents in the 1920s, both in Europe and in the USA. In Europe in particular, doctors were again heavily involved. The first major (i.e. commercially successful in Europe *and* America) instance of what we would now call a European art film is generally agreed to be *The Cabinet of Dr Caligari*,

---

4   Our attitude to neither of these men could be said to constitute trust, however. Both films fall into the somatic horror group.

which was made in Germany by Robert Wiene in 1920. A powerful, dream-like atmosphere pervades this film, as is appropriate for a production that was heavily influenced by the expressionist movement in the arts in Germany at the time. The meaning of the tale – which involves obsessional behaviour, an insane asylum, a carnival sideshow run by a doctor, and a sexually symbolic attraction (yes, just as in *Murders in the Rue Morgue*) – has been the subject of much debate. Was it an allegory about the extreme political danger of institutionalised authority, thus both reflecting and anticipating Germany's travails in the first half of the twentieth century? Or was it the opposite? Did it discredit the supposed heightened awareness of the mentally tortured artist or celebrate it? However, although people argue about what the film means, there is no disagreement that its sets and set-pieces are seminal. The former consisted of painted flats rather than built scenery, their impossible angles and false perspectives amplifying the psychological precariousness of the story; and the latter included scenes that have been replicated a thousand times since – for example, when a threatening figure in black appears at night outside the window of the unprotected heroine.

If *The Cabinet of Dr Caligari* epitomises the generalisation that European horror films of the period were predominantly psychological, then the movies of Lon Chaney well represent America's proclivity for a more physical type of horror. Chaney was celebrated for his ability to radically alter his appearance, his soubriquet *The Man of a Thousand Faces* telling only half the story – his bodily transformations were pretty astonishing, too. Two famous roles were eponymous, namely the phantom of the Opera and the hunchback of Notre Dame; but they had little connection with medicine, so are not within our orbit. *The Unknown* (Browning, 1927) is hardly a medical movie either, but Chaney (as Alonzo, the knife thrower) does require the services of a doctor to perform an unusual kind of cosmetic surgery: he has his arms amputated so that he can win over the woman of his dreams. Even though the woman in question is a very young and beautiful Joan Crawford, this is an extreme recourse. Clearly the logic of the film is bizarre, to put it mildly, and this is not the place to unpick it; but in the context of this chapter, the film usefully illustrates the fact that even when horror is overtly physical, it usually has psychological undercurrents.

So when we reach America in the early 1930s again, by way of our back-track, we have another way of explaining how it came to be a fecund filmic time, because it was the moment when European and American sensibilities really started to come together. This was partly because of the natural spread of ideas in a young and fast-growing field; but also because of an influx of European film-makers who were lured to Hollywood by the time-honoured sibling sirens, Fame and Fortune. The man who directed *Frankenstein* was English (James Whale); the director of *Jekyll and Hyde* was Russian (Rouben Mamoulian), and of course neither source story was American; *Murders in the Rue Morgue* was directed by a Frenchman (Robert Florey), although the (considerably altered) story was written by the American Edgar Allan Poe; and *Island of Lost Souls* was directed by an American (Erle Kenton) while being based on a story of an Englishman (*The Island of Dr Moreau* by HG Wells).

As mentioned earlier, many of these films have been remade, often several times. This suggests that there must be something in them that continues to resonate for audiences, and that there is ground which somehow needs to be covered repeatedly (or at least revisited by each generation). However, if some elements of a remake involve replication, others are more like an update. *Mary Reilly* (Frears, 1996) is a retelling of *Jekyll and Hyde*. It was a critical and box-office failure on release, the wiseacres pointing out that it is the only Julia Roberts film in which she does not smile. However, some movies accrue kudos with the passing of time, and this may prove to be one of them; for Frears never makes an unintelligent film (an early success was *My Beautiful Launderette*; and his most recent one was *The Queen*), and he had the additional fillip on this project of the expert writer Christopher Hampton. Jekyll's activities are here entrenched in the social context of the deplorable double standards and the brutal exercise of masculine power of the Victorian era. Although this angle is not entirely absent from earlier filmic versions – indeed, even Robert Louis Stevenson's original novella hints at it – it is more fully depicted than hitherto, and scenes in a brothel run by Mrs Farraday (played by Glenn Close) are especially chilling. However, what is entirely new is the presence of a maid in the Jekyll household called Mary Reilly, who as the title suggests is the main focus of the film. She is a timid, introverted young Irish woman, who has just been recruited to the domestic staff; and who we discover suffered terrible cruelties as a child at the hands of her father. We watch her evolving relationship with the doctor, her master, and how it gradually extends into his other existence as Hyde; and we see how revulsion vies with attraction in her. If the doctor's self-destructive behaviour appears to be a reaction to the repressive world that he inhabits, Reilly's equivocal response to his perversion of goodness seems to be traceable to childhood trauma – a distressing scenario all round!

However, new medical horror films are not confined to modern reworkings of the classics. Another strand has emerged, concerning films that seem to be made in the realisation that truth is stranger than fiction, and they reopen our inquiry into the enactment of trust. In the films that we have looked at, the main-protagonist doctors have been either partly or wholly evil. It makes a pleasant change, then, to come to Frederick Treves, the doctor who cares for Robert Merrick, the Elephant Man, in the film of that name (Lynch, 1980). This account of (real-life) physical deformity plays like a variation on the Frankenstein story – a normal person is treated abysmally by a brutal society (similar to the fictional world of *Mary Reilly*) because of his appearance, and is paraded at fairs as a freak. The story is filmed not unlike a 1930s horror movie – in black and white, with deep shadows and plenty of cold grey stone – presumably to draw out this parallel. Moreover, David Lynch, the director, appears to have been chosen because of his special feel for unnatural nature – his (only) previous feature film was *Eraserhead* (1977), a surrealist cross between Samuel Beckett and Lon Chaney-type horror involving a foetus. Merrick is a monster in nothing but appearance; and Treves, a doctor, is the first person to realise this. The recognition is not instant, but Treves' compassion and understanding grow as the film progresses. Initially, he too is interested in Merrick only for display purposes, albeit as a living medical specimen rather than a freak show. Thus his shift to benevolence inversely mirrors our previous horror-film doctors' slide in the opposite direction; and conversely it allows Merrick to trust (at least some of) humanity in a way that he has been unable to do before.

The idea of using the cinematic language of horror films when making a film based on true events is also taken up by writer–director Christian de Chalonge in his film *Docteur Petiot* (1990). Marcel Petiot is a doctor who, during World War Two, abuses his position in an almost incredible way. Working as a GP in occupied France, he is shown to be popular with his patients, his outward behaviour (even to his wife and son) suggesting that he is as patriotic and anti-German as it is possible to be without getting into trouble. Accordingly, when he makes it known that he can help Jewish patients to escape from the country, he has no shortage of 'customers.' He asks for money to pay for travel costs and the cooperation of middlemen; and then gets clients to come to his house on the night of their departure to be given final instructions and a false ID. When they arrive, he kills them and disposes of their bodies in the incinerator in the building's cellar. In cahoots with the Gestapo, he receives a share of the estate of his duped, dead, former patients, building up a considerable collection of paintings and statues as well as funds, in which he seems to be largely uninterested. Scenes of him dancing – almost literally – on the graves of his victims are juxtaposed with others where he displays care and consideration towards the living. Very belatedly – several murders into the film (in real life it was after at least 24 murders) – he is arrested and sentenced to death. The film offers no simple explanation for his behaviour, opting instead mainly for detached observation with the occasional subtle suggestion – implying perhaps that such a person is almost beyond comprehension. It is shot in a sepia-tinted colour reminiscent of the German horror films of the 1920s, with several sequences that echo those movies. Petiot (played quite brilliantly by Michel Serrault) is made up to resemble a vampire, to add to the effect. Even more than *The Elephant Man*, this is an out-and-out horror movie that happens to be true. So, although he may not have looked vampiric, we find ourselves back with Harold Shipman; and confronting the sad fact that real-life horrors can exceed anything dreamt up by screenwriters and directors.

Thus medical horror movies give film-makers and audiences the chance to explore a very wide variety of issues. To pick a few examples from the films mentioned, these include cultural tensions relating to the increasing secularisation of life (*Murders in the Rue Morgue*); the collapse of individual sanity and accompanying loss of autonomy (*The Cabinet of Dr Caligari*); the dangerous recourses of a frustrated psyche (*Mary Reilly*). Themes are legion, disparate and complex. They can alter with the *Zeitgeist*, but many recur, implying that they are deep-seated human concerns. Many of them could certainly appear in other genres, and indeed they do, but the horror 'coating' imparts a fearful flavour that seems to hit a certain spot for moviegoers (an excellent academic book about horror has the hard-to-beat title *Dreadful Pleasures*). Of course, many horror movies do not involve doctors; but many do. These films constitute warnings – overstated and unbelievable, perhaps, but real nonetheless.

Further reading
Frayling C. *Mad, Bad and Dangerous? The scientist and the cinema*. London: Reaktion Books; 2005.

Robinson D. *Das Cabinet des Dr Caligari*. BFI Film Classics. London: British Film Institute; 1997.

Twitchell JB. *Dreadful Pleasures: an anatomy of modern horror*. Oxford: Oxford University Press; 1985.

Filmography

MURDERS IN THE RUE MORGUE (1932)

Credits

Director	Robert Florey
Production Company	Universal
Screenplay	Tom Reed, Dale Van Every
Additional Dialogue	John Huston
Original short story	Edgar Allan Poe
Director of Photography	Karl Freund
Editor	Milton Carruth
Art Director	Charles D Hall
Make-up	Jack P Pierce

Cast

Mademoiselle Camille L'Espanaye	Sidney Fox
Doctor Mirakle	Bela Lugosi
Pierre Dupin	Leon Waycoff

ISLAND OF LOST SOULS (1932)

Credits

Director	Erle C Kenton
Production Company	Paramount
Screenplay	Waldemar Young, Philip Wylie
Original novel, *The Island of Dr Moreau*	HG Wells
Director of Photography	Karl Struss
Sound	MM Paggi

Cast

Dr Moreau	Charles Laughton
Sayer of the Law	Bela Lugosi
Edward Parker	Richard Arlen
Ruth Thomas	Leila Hyams
Lota the Panther Woman	Kathleen Burke
Montgomery	Arthur Hohl
M'Ling	Tetsu Komai
Captain Donahue	Paul Hurst

THE CABINET OF DR CALIGARI (1920)

Credits

Director	Robert Wiene
Production Company	Decla Filmgesellschaft
Production	Erich Pommer

Scenario	Carl Mayer, Hans Janowitz
Photography	Willy Hameister
Art Director	Hermann Warm, Walter Reimann,
	Walter Röhrig

Cast

Dr Caligari/director of asylum	Werner Krauss
Cesare	Conrad Veidt
Jane	Lil Dagover
Franzis	Friedrich Feher
Alan	Hans Heinz von Twardowski
Dr Olsen	Rudolf Lettinger

THE UNKNOWN (1927)

Credits

Director	Tod Browning
Production Company	Metro-Goldwyn-Mayer
Scenario	Waldemar Young
Story	Tod Browning
Photography	Merritt B Gerstad
Editor	Harry Reynolds
Art Director	Cedric Gibbons

Cast

Alonzo	Lon Chaney
Jim Malabar	Norman Kerry
Nanon	Joan Crawford
Zanzi	Nick De Ruiz
Cojo	John George
Armless double for Lon Chaney	Dismuki

MARY REILLY (1996)

Credits

Director	Stephen Frears
Production Company	TriStar Pictures
Screenplay	Christopher Hampton
Original novel	Valerie Martin
Director of Photography	Philippe Rousselot
Editor	Lesley Walker
Supervising Art Director	John King
Music	George Fenton

Cast

Mary Reilly	Julia Roberts
Dr Henry Jekyll/Mr Edward Hyde	John Malkovich
Mr Poole	George Cole
Mary's father	Michael Gambon
Mrs Farraday	Glenn Close

THE ELEPHANT MAN (1980)

Credits

Director	David Lynch
Production Company	Brooksfilms
Screenplay	Christopher De Vore, Eric Bergren, David Lynch
Original book	Sir Frederick Treves
Original book	Ashley Montagu
Director of Photography	Freddie Francis
Editor	Anne V Coates
Art Director	Bob Cartwright
Elephant Man make-up	Christopher Tucker
Music	John Morris

Cast

Dr Frederick Treves	Anthony Hopkins
John Merrick	John Hurt
Mrs Madge Kendal	Anne Bancroft
Carr Gomm	John Gielgud
Mothershead	Wendy Hiller
Bytes	Freddie Jones
Night porter	Michael Elphick
Mrs Treves	Hannah Gordon

DOCTEUR PETIOT (1990)

Credits

Director	Christian de Chalonge
Production Company	Sara Films (Paris)
Screenplay	Dominique Garnier, Christian de Chalonge
Director of Photography	Patrick Blossier
Editor	Anita Fernandez
Production Designer	Yves Brover-Rabinovici
Music	Michel Portal

Cast

Docteur Petiot	Michel Serrault
Ivan Drezner	Pierre Romans
Nathan Guzik	Zbigniew Horoks
Georgette Petiot	Bérangère Bonvoisin

CHAPTER 3

Great directors. I: John Ford (1895–1973)

Despite anyone's fond, faint hopes to the contrary, the mainstream US film industry is just that – a mainstream industry. '*Ars gratia artis*' (art for art's sake) reads the Latin logo under the MGM lion, and a full translation into American would surely append the extra phrase 'but money for God's sake.' Why on earth go to all the time, trouble and expense of producing a film if one is not going to make money from it, preferably in large amounts?

However, amidst this general truth lie some contradictions. Small-scale examples come plentifully in the shape of gratuitous (in commercial terms) artfulness of expression – value-adding cinematography can be found in some of the B-est of B-movies.

More significantly, the United State of Hollywood has always contained infiltrators. Admittedly, fifth-column directors have been ruthlessly extirpated upon discovery (Orson Welles is a celebrated example); but some double agents have managed not to blow their cover for an entire career. They somehow contrive to have their cake and eat it – to make commercially successful films within the confines of conventional forms that nonetheless have their own fiercely independent artistic DNA running right through them. These individuals are the so-called auteurs, originally identified and championed as important figures by a group of young French film critics in the 1950s in the face of an indifferent American intelligentsia. In the journal *Cahiers du Cinéma*, the French showed how the films of these men (for Hollywood directors were almost always men), taken singly and as an oeuvre, repaid the most careful consideration; and how said consideration revealed a coherent body of thought akin to that of great artists from more exalted fields, such as literature or painting. At the time, this was a radical proposal; and Irish-American director John Ford was one of their *causes celèbres*.

The contemporary viewer may well have a few things to get past on first meeting Ford. Some of his films come across as mawkishly sentimental, outwardly simplistic and openly patriotic (US-flagwaving-style). However, he was revered by film-makers of many national, political and stylistic hues (as well as the *Cahiers* crowd); and this critical reputation has not diminished since his death – pretty reliable indicators that it is worth looking a little more closely at his movies.

Ford made a lot of Westerns, and they are a good way into his work, not least because they embody the paradox raised in the preceding discussion – that of a populist surface belying artistic depth. The Western is a genre that is often not taken seriously, for obvious reasons. The films traditionally feature goodies and baddies (in white and black hats, respectively) who have punch-ups in saloons (while showgirls look on) and shoot-outs on the street (while timid townspeople take cover). No wonder kids – of all ages – like them. However, Ford imbues his stories of cowboys and indians with closely inter-twined visual and narrative complexity, and a discerning viewer comes away from them with much to ponder on. One of Ford's abiding interests is the history of post-colonial America, a relatively young country whose past does not extend that far back from its present (for example, Ford himself actually met and conversed with Wyatt Earp). In these cowboy films it is as if Ford, like a psychotherapist, is reviewing the nation's childhood in order to better comprehend its adult condition.

The Man Who Shot Liberty Valance (1962) is one of Ford's last films, and a wonderfully mature work. The story is told in flashback (note the link to his-torical enquiry) by a venerable politician (Ransom Stoddard, played by James Stewart) who has greatly advanced the march of progress into cowboy coun-try. His civilising programme has been based on concepts such as lawfulness, statehood, peaceful (if hotly contested) democratic processes, the development of transport infrastructure (in the shape of the railway), and so on. Stoddard has made a special detour on one of his political tours to return to the town where his career started, when he was a young lawyer heading west. Thanks directly and indirectly to him, the town has changed. It now has 'churches, high schools and shops', pillars of orderly socialisation that were notably absent when he originally arrived, borne unconscious by a Good Samaritan, the stagecoach that he was travelling on having been held up, after which he was beaten and left for dead by the brutal Liberty Valance. Stoddard and his wife have now come to attend the funeral of the Good Samaritan, although we do not see the funeral or even discover how the man died. Instead, the film's narrative climbs in through the small window between someone's death and their burial, when that person can still seem almost alive even as we come to terms with their death – an interim when profound reflection (in this case on the part of Stoddard and his wife) is stirred up and has not yet crystallised into fixed memory.

In the flashback, which occupies all but the first and last few minutes of the film, we watch a story unfold that encapsulates the taming of the Wild West; and it is a story that contains a degree of ambivalence, or at least an acknowledgement of the regrettable losses that sometimes accompany desirable gains. Not only are the events themselves tinged with complexity, but so is their recording. In a post-flashback scene, the town's newspaperman is presented with the chance to correct the history books, Stoddard having given a first-hand account for the first time. He eschews the opportunity, uttering one of the great movie quotes to explain his decision: 'This is the West, sir. When the legend becomes fact, print the legend.' It's a statement that renders the film's title at once ironic and narratively subversive, as those who watch it will see; and it points up a frightening American tendency to embrace myth rather than truth.

(The movie also deals in another kind of mythology. James Stewart's best-known cinematic persona is the incarnation of benign, liberal American values – it is a role that he has played over and over again in various contexts. Ford exploits this pre-established, emblematic status by putting it in the ring and letting it fight it out with a contrasting, equally recognisable cinematic archetype, that of John Wayne. Wayne's stock personality – fast on the draw, slow on the drawl – is also deployed purposefully. So in part *The Man Who Shot Liberty Valance* is a film about the clash between American cinematic myths, with Stewart as the peaceful champion of the ordinary guy, and Wayne as the righter-of-wrongs man of action. Both are forces for good, and both are etched deep as ideal types in America's sense of positive self-image. Ford's degree of self-consciousness (of which any Modernist author would have been proud) is also evident in the filmic legerdemain used to pull off the film title's conceit. As in all great art, form and content are inseparable.)

Among the locals whom we meet in the course of the flashback is a doctor, whose status in the town is marginal. His main function seems to be to act as an (excess) drinking companion to the editor of the local paper (who plays a much more important role), and to pronounce people dead. He is referred to from time to time, in distinctly unawed terms ('Go find Doc Willoughby – if he's sober, bring him back'); and although *ipso facto* meriting inclusion in the story (otherwise he would not have been in the screenplay), he is an onlooker rather than an active protagonist.

By contrast, the doctor in *Stagecoach* (1939) has a major supporting part. He is more than drunk most of the time – he is an unabashed alcoholic, who is being kicked out of town for non-payment of rent. However, his parlous condition, although it is given no backstory, seems to be a by-product of his sensibility – he quotes the classics as if he understands them, and is very observant of nuances of human interaction. His (very temporary) sobering up is important to the story at one point, as is his presence during the climactic shoot-out.

Stagecoach has a blue-chip origin in the shape of a celebrated Maupassant short story called 'Boule de Suif' (which did not include a doctor), although it seems that Ford discovered it via an intermediary source. Maupassant's story concerned a disparate group of people who set off on a coach journey which is then beset by difficulties; and the film is so loose an adaptation that any comparisons are redundant, but one thing is worth noting here: Ford (and his scriptwriter Dudley Nichols) have taken on Maupassant's great economy and acuity, assembling and sketching the small band of protagonists quickly and brilliantly. In this regard, the doctor has a special and subtle function, acting virtually as a disinterested conscience for the group even as he is in the process of capitulating to his own flaws.

Stagecoach is by common consent one of the key works in the cinematic canon. In it, Ford virtually invented the idea of the grown-up Western, not to mention redefining the art of location shooting and editing. It has an opening shot worthy of an Impressionist painter, consisting of a vast expanse of sun-baked scrubland with mountains in the distance, and no evidence of human presence whatsoever apart from a rough mud road that comes into the frame diagonally from the bottom right-hand corner and has disappeared into the scrub before it gets to the centre. Much of the film is shot in the now iconic, but at the time never previously filmed (and of course totally tarmac-free) Monument Valley. This is pioneer country, and *Stagecoach* is not only set *in* the landscape, but it is also *about* it, the 'geography is destiny' idea being brought vividly to life.

Our reverse-chronology interest in some of Ford's doctors leads us back to three films that he made in the 1930s which had physicians at their epicentre, namely *Prisoner of Shark Island* (1936), *Doctor Bull* (1933) and *Arrowsmith* (1931), his excellent filmic rendition of the classic medical *Bildungsroman*.

The first of these films is apparently most closely linked to *Stagecoach* and *The Man Who Shot Liberty Valance* by historical setting, because it also takes place in the Old West. However, it in fact relates as much to the period in which it was made as to the period in which it was set; and its closest relation in the Ford canon is probably the more famous *The Grapes of Wrath* (1940).

It is the true story of Dr Samuel Mudd, a country doctor who tends the damaged leg of a man who arrives on his doorstep one stormy night (on 15 April 1865, to be precise), and so helps him to continue his journey. Mudd has no idea who the man is, but we viewers do; for we have just seen him assassinate Abraham Lincoln in a theatre in Washington, and injure a leg during his getaway. The next day, troops arrest Mudd; and he is tried for complicity in the assassination. The trial is a military rather than a civil one, because of the extremity of the crime and the state of martial law that exists in the aftermath of the recently ended Civil War. The attorney general gives the adjudicating military officers clear instructions – the precarious state of the Union and the bloodlust of an outraged population require that they must overlook 'trifling technicalities' of law and 'pedantic regard for customary rules of evidence, especially the concept of reasonable doubt.' Mudd is duly found guilty, and in the course of the trial we see how a little circumstantial evidence and a prevailing moral climate can turn right-thinking individuals into agents of injustice. It is a point that is made repeatedly throughout the film. Just as in the immediate aftermath of the assassination, we the audience are party to information (about Mudd's innocence) that most of the characters on screen are not. This is a classic narrative strategy – think of Hitchcock's 'wrong man' films such as *The 39 Steps* (1935) – which has the effect of closely allying us to Mudd himself, who is now of course also 'in the know.' At times we want to shout at the screen 'It's unfair – he acted in ignorance!', just as Mudd does to the string of people who treat him as a hateful traitor, for Lincoln was much loved. Our impotence and frustration are (miniature) forms of his.

Mudd is sent to Shark Island, a prison just off the coast of Florida where living conditions are extremely harsh and the guards' behaviour is even harsher. Here he modifies his hitherto passive stance (his implicit acceptance of the state's right to do as it sees fit to individuals) and tries to escape. He fails, and is confined in a lightless pen underground. It is at this point, just when it seems that all hope has died, that he is given a rope to pull himself back up into the land of the living; and this rope is his medical knowledge.[5] An outbreak of yellow fever has decimated the occupants of the island – prisoners and warders – and the commandant is at his wits' end, because the prison doctor (who has been portrayed equivocally) has also succumbed to the disease. In desperation, the commandant asks Mudd for help; and Mudd accedes unhesitatingly, with a reply as momentous as it is pithy: 'Once before, I was a doctor. I'm still a doctor.' The two sentences show that he is unrepentant – he feels that he did no wrong in helping a man in need before – and that he believes his professional mantle must sit over his personal clothing. He brings the disease under control; and thereby engineers his own social redemption (he is pardoned in the light of his near-heroic medical deeds) as well as the correction of a grave societal error (his imprisonment). So it is that he acts as a healing agent for a society that has damaged itself, doing so by holding on to his own virtues in the face of enormous tribulations. (A remake today might be called '*Prisoner of Robben Island*' or '*Prisoner of Guantanamo Bay*.') Ford's contention appears to be that individual idealism is the only possible lifeboat when the ship is going down;[6] and in this instance that idealism is enshrined in the Hippocratic Oath.

Historians now question the extent of Mudd's innocence, with the consensus seeming to be that it was partial at best. For instance, he had in fact met Booth the assassin several times before the event, and was a known pro-South agitator. This makes some of the factual detail of the film entirely untrue; but it does not, I think, reduce its power one iota. Nor do the handful of unlikely and undeniably corny scenes (and this applies to the other Ford films we have looked at) – if one takes all of these elements to be symbolic rather than realistic, they work fine. For instance, the prison sergeant (played almost satanically by John Carradine), who has been most vigorous in his dislike of Mudd, is the first to shake Mudd's hand when his reputation is rehabilitated. Granted, the sergeant's was the first life that Mudd had saved (a too obvious

---

5   It is ironic but surely not coincidental that it was precisely his medical knowledge that had landed him in his current predicament.

6   The metaphor conveniently allows me to make a trivial point. Mudd's wife is played by the luminous Gloria Stuart, who appeared in the blockbusting *Titanic* (1997) over 60 years later. Unsurprisingly, she was the only member of the cast of that film who had been alive at the time of the actual nautical disaster.

set-up); but it remains a highly implausible volte-face. Yet if the viewer sees this as signifying an end of polarised conflict and hatred; and a beginning of rapprochement and reintegration; then although it may be optimistic it is not incredible. Another caveat is that the representation of Afro-Americans in the movie is sometimes offensively dated. (Although it is not always so – Mudd's film-long relationship with the black man who works his estate is far from simply racist.)

The story seems to me to be partly about the legacy of profound civil unrest (in this case, the American Civil War), both the distorting effect it has on people's behaviour and the consequent damage that it wreaks on individuals and the state. It is also about the lived experience of that legacy. I mentioned at the start that the film had one foot in the period in which it was made, and transposing the message to the 1930s, it fits into a genre of social conscience movies that painted a grim picture of the Depression, and little people's impotence in the face of big social forces that were running out of control. It is not by chance that the start of the film has an intertitle of a signed message about political revisionism from the then (Democratic) Senator for Maryland.

Finally, it would be a criminal act almost on the scale of Lincoln's assassination not to mention the extraordinary cinematography of the film. The lighting-cameraman Bert Glennon (who also worked on *Stagecoach*) surpassed himself in the thrilling attempted-escape sequence, as well as the chiaroscuro shots in Mudd's cell, which bring Goya to mind. It is a feast for the eyes, and enhances the film greatly.

The apogee of this chapter might have been *Arrowsmith* (a film that received four Oscar nominations and was Ford's first box-office smash), but it isn't. Despite a beginning (featuring a wagon train heading west and a determined pioneer) that appears to locate us bang in the middle of the Ford territory which we have been exploring, the story soon moves on to different pastures. As such it is less interesting in the context of this chapter, for it is a young work, in which Ford seems sometimes to be dominated by his material. This is perhaps unsurprising, given that the source novel by Sinclair Lewis had won the Pulitzer Prize. If the viewer who has read the novel cannot but mourn the loss of Lewis' wonderful prose, the film nonetheless does a pretty good job of getting the book on to the screen, incorporating a raft of issues (including important explorations of scientific research ethics) in under 90 minutes. Moreover, it still gives ample evidence of Ford's own prodigious talent (one short sequence in which the eponymous hero contemplates starting an affair is filmed particularly nicely), as well as hints of Fordian themes to come. So, taken on its own, it is a rich and fascinating movie that deserves attention.[7]

Filmography

ARROWSMITH (1931)

Credits

Director	John Ford
Production	Samuel Goldwyn Inc./John Ford
Screenplay	Sidney Howard
Original novel	Sinclair Lewis
Photography	Ray June
Editor	Hugh Bennett
Sets	Richard Day
Musical score	Alfred Newman

Cast

Dr Martin Arrowsmith	Ronald Colman
Leora Tozer Arrowsmith	Helen Hayes
Professor Max Gottlieb	AE Anson
Gustav Sondelius	Richard Bennett
Joyce Lanyon	Myrna Loy
Dr Oliver Marchand	Clarence Brooks

THE PRISONER OF SHARK ISLAND (1936)

Credits

Director	John Ford
Production Company	Twentieth Century Fox Film Corporation
Screenplay	Nunnally Johnson
From the life story of	Dr Samuel A Mudd
Photography	Bert Glennon
Editor	Jack Murray
Art Director	William Darling
Music Director	Louis Silvers

Cast

Dr Samuel Alexander Mudd	Warner Baxter
Mrs Peggy Mudd	Gloria Stuart
Buckland Montmorency 'Buck' Tilford	Ernest Whitman

---

7 As does *Doctor Bull*, a Ford film from 1933. This is set in contemporary rather than olden days, and is currently hard to obtain on DVD; and so has not been discussed here.

Commandant of Fort Jefferson	Harry Carey
Colonel Dyer	Claude Gillingwater
Doctor MacIntyre	OP Heggie
Sergeant Rankin	John Carradine
John Wilkes Booth	Francis McDonald

STAGECOACH (1939)

Credits

Director	John Ford
Production Company	Walter Wanger Productions
Released through	United Artists
Screenplay	Dudley Nichols
Original story	Ernest Haycox
Director of Photography	Bert Glennon
Film Editor	Dorothy Spencer
Art Director	Alexander Toluboff
Musical Director	Boris Morros

Cast

Dallas	Claire Trevor
The Ringo Kid	John Wayne
Buck Rickabaugh, stagecoach driver	Andy Devine
Marshal Curley Wilcox	George Bancroft
Hatfield	John Carradine
Doc Josiah Boone	Thomas Mitchell
Lucy Mallory	Louise Platt
Samuel Peacock	Donald Meek
Henry Gatewood	Berton Churchill

THE MAN WHO SHOT LIBERTY VALANCE (1962)

Credits

Director	John Ford
Production Company	Paramount Pictures Corporation/John Ford Productions
Screenplay	James Warner Bellah, Willis Goldbeck
Original story	Dorothy M Johnson
Director of Photography	William H Clothier
Editor	Otho Lovering
Art Director	Hal Pereira, Eddie Imazu
Set Decoration	Sam Comer, Darrell Silvera
Music	Cyril Mockridge

Cast

Tom Doniphon	John Wayne
Ransom Stoddard	James Stewart
Hallie Stoddard	Vera Miles
Liberty Valance	Lee Marvin
Pompey	Woody Strode
Dutton Peabody	Edmond O'Brien
Doc Willoughby	Ken Murray
Link Appleyard	Andy Devine
Starbuckle	John Carradine
Nora Erickson	Jeanette Nolan
Peter Erickson	John Qualen

Destination: out?

Assuming they have any choice in the matter, it might appear that people decamp to foreign climes for all sorts of reasons, but perhaps there are only really two – to run away from something they know too well, or to run towards something they think they want to know better. So a film that accompanies them to pastures new has an obvious and almost irresistible starting point: are their hopes met or dashed? However, such films often also have a more outward-looking aspect: what sort of place have these voyagers in fact come to? The main protagonists, acting as surrogates for us cinema-goers, enter a new and usually very different world. They are strangers in a strange land, and their fresh eyes see with a clarity that comes from lack of familiarity and (at least initially) disinterest. This builds an implicit balance-sheet enquiry into the film: is the new environment good or bad? The research is carried out qualitatively using participant observation!

How do these kinds of stories play themselves out when they have a doctor at their centre? For while travellers may take sundry baggage with them, a doctor's luggage always seems to include a medical bag, whether he or she likes it or not. Using five films set in different times and places, this chapter will explore these issues and some matters arising.

Crisis (Brooks, 1950)

The first of the films opens with the main character-cum-medic on vacation[8] in an unnamed Latin American country, the sort of place that used to be called a banana republic, and for which the phrase 'politically volatile' might have

---

8 Because he is on holiday, the doctor needs no backstory. Consequently, the biographical (inward-looking) element of his voyage of discovery is reduced.

been coined. He and his wife decide to beat a hasty retreat after they find themselves too close for comfort to a revolutionist's bomb blast. However, they are whisked from their car at a road-block and 'escorted' (by armed guards) to the presidential quarters, where the doctor's services are required – for the doctor turns out to be Dr Eugene Ferguson, a Johns Hopkins man and world-famous surgeon; and the president has a brain tumour.[9] Soon the two men find themselves embroiled in the ongoing dialogue (or debate) that is at the heart of the film. The president (a military dictator) sees strength, often expressed brutally, as the key component of leadership; and leadership as the key to successful management of his country. The doctor is appalled at this *modus operandi*, his liberal-consensual sensibilities offended; and he says as much, articulately: 'The choice [to come to attend the president] wasn't mine. I dislike force of any kind by anybody.' The president, just as articulately, scoffs at his naivety, arguing that the doctor's ignorance of local history invalidates his pampered philosophy. An early scene is a classic in the doctors-in-film oeuvre. The president is a man who takes orders from no one, not even his wife (a formidable operator in her own right, in marked contrast to Mrs Ferguson, who is missing her shopping on Fifth Avenue). He has had Ferguson (already somewhat vulnerable, being far from home) delivered to him, and is well aware that the doctor will have to treat him because of the medical oath. He holds the whip hand and he knows it. And yet this position of towering supremacy is instantaneously reversed when Ferguson starts to act professionally (i.e. in his capacity as a doctor rather than a tourist). He has the room emptied of sundry colonels and flunkies; he examines the president moderately invasively (with an optoscope); he unhesitatingly tells him what to do ('Raise your arms, please. Now close your eyes'), and the president obediently does his bidding, just like any other patient. The doctor even induces a mild seizure as part of his differential diagnosis without any fear of retribution. By dint of the examination, he shows the president the severity of his condition in a manner that is as humbling as it is irrefutable. It would be hard to better this as a demonstration of sapiental power in action; and hard to think – in the modern, secular world – of anyone apart from a doctor who could provide it. For his part, the doctor has to wrestle with the ethics of saving the life of a man who he thinks is morally objectionable to the point of being evil, and whose position gives him power to harm an entire population.

---

9 It is a mark of this film's overall quality that the fact that the brain surgeon is acted by Cary Grant in no way strains the credibility.

As a point of passing interest, there is the background presence of a (sympathetic) American who works for an oil company, and is a self-proclaimed 'sort of unofficial US ambassador out here.' At one point the president, seeking some tangible (i.e. financial) support in dealing with increasingly widespread insurgency, reminds the man that 'Your company has made millions out of this country!' However, the oil company worker demurs, stating plainly 'You know my hands are tied.' Although not at all trite, this is perhaps the only scene that seems dated now. How perceptions of multinational corporations and political machinations have changed!

Windom's Way (Neame, 1958)

This film has an extraordinary start: the burly man beats the Rank Films gong as per usual, and then for the best part of two minutes much is said – but not a single word is in English. We are witnessing the immediate aftermath of a happy birth, and the presiding doctor exchanging comments with the mother and a small crowd of delighted onlookers in the hut where the event has taken place. His dress and skin colour mark him out as different to the locals, who appear to be Indonesian; but there is no other way of telling that he is British until he finally says something in English to a local nurse – although the fact that he is played by Peter Finch[10] would have left a contemporary audience in little doubt as to his nationality. This introduction is in marked contrast to most other 'Westerners abroad' films, which invariably include a scene where the Western-world newcomer is bewildered at being excluded from understanding what is going on around him because it is being talked about in a language other than English. It is a daring opening gambit by the film-maker, because of its potentially alienating effect on the audience, who are the only ones excluded; and it serves to emphasise the extent to which the doctor has merged into local society as well as the primacy – and hence respect – that this (First World) film intends to accord the (Third World) culture in which it is set.[11]

Finch is the eponymous Windom, a man who personifies a certain post-war British ideal – a doctor who is pragmatic yet idealistic, selfless yet far from self-effacing, skilled, good-natured if sometimes headstrong, good-looking in a careless kind of way, and the list of attractive attributes goes on. He has

---

10 Finch was a well-known leading man of English films in the 1950s.
11 This is also the only film among our quintet in which the expat doctor does not go 'home' at the end – a further sign of its resistance of cliché.

chosen, it transpires, to expatriate himself in order to distance himself from his beautiful upper-class wife and her social set. (In the course of the film she comes out to fetch him; and learns, the hard way, about her limitations before transcending them and forming a new type of relationship with her husband.)

Because his profession simultaneously gives him an intimate involvement with local society and a multilaterally recognised neutrality, Windom finds himself drawn deeper and deeper into ever more fractious industrial relations, with the government and the local rubber plantation owner on one side, and the villagers on the other (with the lurking presence of armed communist rebels in the hills). The film is notable for its steadfast avoidance of judgements – right and wrong are shared out fairly evenly, rather as in real life – for which one imagines praise is due to the screenplay of Jill Craigie, an accomplished writer and film-maker (and wife of Labour party stalwart Michael Foot). At any rate, the doctor's position as a self-appointed mediator becomes increasingly untenable. Events overtake him, and he comes to realise, painfully, that he has overreached himself and ought to have followed the advice he was given earlier in the film to 'stick to doctoring.' His realisation is equally deflating for the audience, given the values that he embodies. He has done nothing reproachable, so the film is not a simple cautionary tale. Rather, it is a sobering observation in the tradition of the great humanist film-makers about the way of the world, and man's limited ability to control it. Although it is played out in a remote territory, it seems probable that Windom – because of his nature – would have had a similar experience wherever he was based. Certainly, 50 years after its release, the film still stands as an exceptionally thoughtful exploration of the dilemmas of a community medic.

City of Joy (Joffé, 1992)

By the time he made *City of Joy*, director-producer Roland Joffé's CV already included *The Killing Fields* (1984) and *The Mission* (1986), two films that expressed outrage at the social injustices being perpetrated at particular historical moments in distant lands. In *City of Joy*, he retains an 'exotic' setting (modern-day Calcutta replaces Cambodia and eighteenth-century South America, respectively) but tempers his strident approach a little. The film is dedicated to Mother Teresa, which suggests that Joffé believes stoicism can sometimes be as heroic as fighting (not that the visceral element is absent – there are scenes involving quite distressing violence).

Unsurprisingly, given its dedicatee, a female nurse is a key figure; but it is perhaps a mark of the film's limited ambition that the part is played by a white English actress of the feisty but ultimately house-trained variety in the shape of Pauline Collins. Furthermore, the nurse plays second fiddle to a self-absorbed American doctor who comes to India to escape feelings of guilt after a child dies at his hands on the operating table. (More negative kudos also accretes because of the casting of American would-be handsome leading man Patrick Swayze as the doctor.) The story all too obviously pits these protagonists against the myriad problems of the city slums as they try to bring health and happiness to the local population. The doctor gradually exchanges self-pity for committed social activism – a storyline that is more of a cheap package holiday than a voyage of discovery. These caveats aside, there are things to admire in the film, and it retains a certain emotional power despite its use of somewhat devalued currency. At times it conveys the genuine miseries of life lived in poverty, and shows the social degeneration that can feed off them – for instance, gangsters who start small but end up having chains of command that reach far up the social ladder. Significantly, change is seen as being rooted in collective action as much as in individual choice; and the doctor is not valorised (much) more than he needs to be.

The Last King of Scotland (Macdonald, 2006)

The Last King of Scotland might almost be an amalgamation of our first three movies, and a corny one at that. It is the story of a newly qualified Scottish medical graduate who, desperate to avoid the stultifying prospect of inheriting his doctor-father's family practice, sticks a pin in the atlas and thereby selects a country in which to do work of the 'Médecins Sans Frontières' type. By a further combination of chance and whimsy, he is almost instantly appointed as personal physician of that country's president; and is soon implicated in political events far outside his frame of reference. On paper, then, this well-trodden plot might not hold much appeal if you have seen the other films discussed. On celluloid, however, it is brimful of an energy that brushes aside any concerns about lack of originality after the first few minutes.

The film hinges on a bold (although not unprecedented, and subsequently increasingly popular) narrative premise – that it is possible to mix fact and fiction without compromising either. Nicholas Garrigan, the young doctor, is a fabrication, lightly but credibly sketched against a social backdrop of the early 1970s. The president is Idi Amin (recreated in a tour-de-force and Oscar-winning performance by American actor Forest Whitaker), who has just come to power in Uganda on a wave of popularity. From this set-up, the film constructs a surprisingly plausible scenario whereby Garrigan, despite his youth and reticence, becomes an important influence on affairs of state. We understand and sympathise a little with him at the start of the film. He is just another young, middle-class man in search of a way to cut loose and assert his own identity; he may be a little selfish, and mildly unprincipled when it comes to sexual mores, but only to a degree that is well within the bounds of acceptability for most 23-year-olds in this country. The film repeatedly shows that he is not fundamentally irresponsible or uncaring – quite the contrary – and indeed it is his likeableness that makes the way the story unfolds so unsettling. For by a series of small, almost unwitting steps he moves from relative innocence to relative guilt. As a direct result of his (non-medical) actions, people suffer and die. The consequences of his deeds are brought home to him most forcefully, causing him considerable psychological and ultimately physical pain. This is certainly not the rite of passage he was hoping for. And for the audience, too, the story proves to be a very harrowing one – which is entirely appropriate, given the real-life component of its subject matter.

Dirty Pretty Things (Frears, 2002)

It would be nice and neat if the films cited so far could be taken as a longitudinal cinematic survey, the subject of which was the growing post-war awareness of the complexity of the relationship between the western world (of which medicine is a powerful symbol) and developing countries. After all, the history is logged by the films in roughly 10-year chunks (1950, 1958, 1971[12] and 1992); and the geography covers four corners of the Earth (Latin America, the East Indies, Africa and Asia). This line of thought makes one want to complete the set by uncovering a film from the 1980s set in, say, Australia. However, the purpose of this chapter is not to try to impose a linear structure, but rather to draw attention to films that are more or less timeless – which is a reasonable (if inevitably subjective) indication of artistic if not sociological merit. And in fact our films do not so much show a development as offer a series of different takes on a set of themes, the earliest having as much to say to a contemporary audience as the most recent.

Notwithstanding all of this, our last film does confer a certain, perhaps fragile, tidiness on the chapter in that it brings us to the here and now. It was

---

12 *The Last King of Scotland* was of course made 35 years after the period in which it was set, and is the only non-contemporaneous film in our group.

made in the last 10 years, and takes place in present-day England. From a British perspective, then, the issues of the previous films are played out in reverse. This film is about immigrants, not emigrants; and the camera lens is now acting as a mirror rather than a telescope. That inversion is reinforced by a change of social scale. Unlike *Crisis*, *Windom's Way* and *The Last King of Scotland*, which deal with high-profile events involving presidents and large-scale upheaval, *Dirty Pretty Things* involves people who are small to the point of near-invisibility (as is explicitly stated at one point near the end of the film), and it looks from the bottom up at a mainstream world with which we are all familiar – or rather, half-familiar.

Okwe ekes out an existence as a desk clerk in a central London hotel by night and a minicab driver by day. He is also an illegal immigrant from Nigeria and a doctor who, it emerges, is wanted for murder in his own country. Each of these five social identities contributes significantly to his story; but the medical one turns out to be of paramount importance, at least when it comes to pulling the plot together.

With acute observation and plenty of human detail, the film paints a picture of the many invidious side-effects of our prosperous, mock-socialist, capitalist society, as played out through its multi-subcultural black economy. The ultimate incarnation (literally) of this is the market in illegal organ sale, whereby people 'swap their insides for a passport.' Okwe's medical background takes him, reluctantly, into the midst of this twenty-first-century equivalent of the slave trade; but it also gives him the means of mounting a counter-attack. (To say more would spoil the film for those who have not seen it.) Moreover, his training brings him benefits in other ways (for instance, it is instrumental in his forging many mutually supportive relationships throughout the film). However, although medicine sucks him into some situations that he does not like and others that he does, it remains a tool, for it is Okwe's mindset – his belief system, his values, his day-to-day comportment – that ultimately defines him, not his professional qualification. And the film shares this important, implicit premise with all the others discussed in this chapter.

Movies that feature doctors abroad prove to be very good vehicles for exploring several substantial themes. One of these is the collision between individual lives and the societies in which they are lived – a fusion of the two points raised at the start of this chapter. A new arrival in a culture offers film-makers a point of departure into that culture, and a pretext to take a tour of the parts of it that they feel to be of note. A doctor is particularly useful for this.

Because of his professional attributes and social position, he is a ready-made (even codified) passepartout, who necessitates few implausible additions to the storyline, as anyone can get sick and call for a doctor. (Of course, calling for a doctor does not necessarily mean that the sick person will comply with the doctor's advice – a fact that creates the further narrative possibility of a power struggle.)

If these films deal with movement in and out of a culture, could we draw a parallel between doctors' movement in and out of patients' lives? After all, in the first consultation a clinician moves from ignorance of to intimacy with (and implication in) a patient's life in an unnaturally short space of time. And what of the issue of emotional distance? Is there something to be said here about the 'correct' degree of professional detachment? In our films, there is certainly a recurrent tension between the medical requirement to get involved and the concomitant professional need to maintain neutrality. (They generally appear to take the line that doctors should stay away from the body politic and stick to the body human.)

Another even more symbolic line of enquiry would be to ask how the intrinsic professional detachment of being a medic relates to the narratives of physical detachment of our expatriates. That approach would equate 'home' with subjective/personal existence, and 'abroad' with the objective/ patient world; doctor–patient interaction becoming the journey between the two. However, the runway for this discussion runs out before we can achieve take-off; because our films do not even ask let alone answer this question, preferring to concentrate on the social dimensions of their stories rather than those relating solely to medical practice. (Have we identified a gap in the canon here?)

This chapter has looked at cultural juxtapositions in relation to journeys of significant distance. However, in many parts of the UK, especially in the multicultural metropolises, there are of course countless 'foreign' cultures all around all the time, which makes everyone both an insider and an outsider. So these films might be telling us home truths as well as 'away' ones (indeed, this is one of the 'messages' of *Dirty Pretty Things*). And, come to think of it, are we not all strangers in strange lands when it comes to encounters with other people?

Filmography

DIRTY PRETTY THINGS (2002)

Credits

Director	Stephen Frears
Production Companies	BBC Films, Miramax
Screenplay	Steven Knight
Photography	Chris Menges
Editor	Mick Audsley
Music	Nathan Larson

Cast

Okwe	Chiwetel Ejiofor
Senay	Audrey Tautou
Juan (Sneaky)	Sergi Lopez
Juliette	Sophie Okonedo
Guo Yi	Benedict Wong
Ivan	Zlatko Buric

WINDOM'S WAY (1958)

Credits

Director	Ronald Neame
Production Company	Rank Film Productions
Script	Jill Craigie
Original novel	James Ramsey Ullman
Photography	Christopher Challis
Editor	Reginald Mills
Music	James Bernard

Cast

Dr Alec Windom	Peter Finch
Lee Windom	Mary Ure
Anna Vidal	Natasha Parry
George Hasbrook	Robert Flemyng
Patterson	Michael Hordern
Jan Vidal	John Cairney

CRISIS (1950)

Credits

Director	Richard Brooks
Production Company	Metro-Goldwyn-Mayer
Producer	Arthur Freed
Script	Richard Brooks

Original story	George Tabori
Photography	Ray June
Editor	Robert J Kern
Art Director	Cedric Gibbons
Music	Miklós Rozsa

Cast

Dr Eugene Ferguson	Cary Grant
Raoul Farrago	José Ferrer
Isabel Farrago	Signe Hasso
Helen Ferguson	Paula Raymond

CITY OF JOY (1992)

Credits

Director	Roland Joffé
Production Company	TriStar Pictures
Screenplay	Mark Medoff
Original novel	Dominique Lapierre
Photography Director	Peter Biziou

Cast

Dr Max Lowe	Patrick Swayze
Hasari Pal	Om Puri
Joan Bethel	Pauline Collins
Kamla Pal	Shabana Azmi
Amrita Pal	Ayesha Dharkar
Shambu Pal	Santu Chowdhury
Manooj Pal	Imran Badsah Khan
Ashoka	Art Malik

THE LAST KING OF SCOTLAND (2006)

Credits

Director	Kevin Macdonald
Production companies	DNA Films Ltd, Channel Four Television Corporation
Screenplay	Peter Morgan, Jeremy Brock
Original novel	Giles Foden
Director of Photography	Anthony Dod Mantle
Editor	Justine Wright
Production Designer	Michael Carlin
Music	Alex Heffes

Cast

Idi Amin	Forest Whitaker
Dr Nicholas Garrigan	James McAvoy
Kay Amin	Kerry Washington
Stone	Simon McBurney
Dr Junju	David Oyelowo
Dr Merrit	Adam Kotz
Sarah Merrit	Gillian Anderson
Jonah Wasswa	Stephen Rwangyezi
Masanga	Abby Mukiibi

CHAPTER 5

Visuality: mapping the overlap

Doctors have always made use of the five senses in pursuit of their work. Taste is not high in the hit parade these days, but used to be called upon to diagnose sick babies (a salty forehead augured ill!); smell has also fallen out of favour, but is still used to detect possible renal failure. Touch, of course, remains an integral part of everyday practice in many specialties. Probably the two most commonly employed senses are sight and hearing. Notwithstanding the enormous iconic power of the stethoscope, and the sundry bodily murmurings that doctors heed, the single most important sound that is heard is undoubtedly patients' utterances. However, the realm of the visual is much more diverse, and is evolving constantly, both in scientific observation in general and in medicine in particular. Medicine uses a variety of more or less invasive scans and scopes: X-rays and MRIs are examples of the former; and microscopes, endoscopes and arthroscopes are examples of the latter. A close study of the history of biotechnology and its relationship to the clinical gaze can be found in Lisa Cartwright's book *Screening the Body: tracing medicine's visual culture* (Cartwright, 1995). Continuing to work from the inside of the body out, using only the naked eye, doctors often examine patients' outer layer, namely the skin, not to mention their general demeanour (the non-verbal cues).

Meanwhile, cinema works its wonders to perform through only two senses, sight and sound[13] – the same pair that we have highlighted as most pertinent to modern medicine, a similarity that constitutes one of the two coincidences that lie at the heart of this book. Again sound, especially speech, is crucial, and we downplay it at our peril; but in origin cinema is a visual

---

13 As if to prove this point, *Sight and Sound* is the name of the British Film Institute's monthly journal.

medium. Indeed, purists argue that *le septième Art* ('the seventh art', as the French dubbed it early on) reached its pinnacle with the golden silents of the 1920s, because the arrival of dialogue (which accompanied the introduction of sound) at the end of that decade completely reoriented it, bringing it much closer to theatre and reducing its reliance on pure visuality.[14] And if the silent era was when cinema was perhaps most unlike any other art form, then it was certainly the time when the ground rules were laid down for what still comprises the language of film.

This language can be divided into four categories. The first is the shot, which is the basic component of filming, since it is most closely tied to the camera. A shot begins when the camera operator presses down the button that makes the instrument work, and finishes when he lifts his finger off the button. Shots are described according to their framing (whether they are close-ups, or extreme long shots, or whatever – essentially a description of how far the camera is away from the subject that it is filming); their angle (e.g. low-angle, overhead); and their movement (e.g. pans, tilts, dollies[15] in or out, etc.).

Next comes editing, which involves joining together the strips of film from different shots to make a whole movie. Crudely speaking, there are two schools of thought about the philosophy of editing. The first of these, developed by Russian film-makers such as Sergei Eisenstein in the silent era, saw editing as the distinguishing feature of film as an art. They felt that, uniquely in cinema, meaning could be built up by the juxtaposition of images which created a meta-meaning transcending that of the images in isolation (i.e. the total could be greater than the sum of the parts). The Kuleshov experiment – so often cited that one almost feels it must be apocryphal! – 'proved' their point. People were asked to interpret a series of shots of a man's face intercut with different images. He looked hungry, they said, when the preceding shot was of a bowl of soup; 'Now he looks sad!' they agreed, when the previous shot was of a woman in a coffin; and so on. Of course, the film-maker used an identical shot of the man on each occasion!

If it had been left there, the so-called Kuleshov effect would have been just another 'A'-level-psychology-type experiment; but it was harnessed – along with close attention to the rhythm of image juxtaposition – to the

---

14 This time it was the Americans who came up with an appropriate new name – 'the talkies.'

15 A dolly is a platform on wheels that allows a camera to move around smoothly. These days, zoom lenses and lighter 'steadicams' allow film-makers to achieve similar effects, which is particularly useful when shooting in real-life locations.

greater goal of creating a new way of conveying complex messages, and the Russians explored it in classics of the film canon such as *Battleship Potemkin* (Eisenstein, 1925). (This style of editing is referred to as montage.)

Meanwhile, a very different approach to editing also developed – editing which sought not to celebrate but to conceal itself. This style, which was referred to as 'continuity editing' and was embraced by Hollywood, tried to make the transition from one shot to another as smooth as possible, in order to minimise the threat to the spectator's suspension of disbelief. Thus when we see an actor walk up to a door and open it, the next shot will often be of the door viewed from the other side opening and the actor appearing from behind it. The viewer then links the two shots, inferring cause and effect – because of the so-called 'match-on-action' cut. Of course, the second shot may have been filmed several weeks after the first, and it may not even have been the same door! Another common ploy is called the 'point of view cut.' Here a close-up of an actor, staring at something out of the frame and usually emoting fiercely, is followed by a shot of the thing (we deduce) that he is looking at from his point of view. The effect of this one-two is to activate viewers' empathy, although on the briefest reflection the artificiality of the set-up is apparent. There are several of these standard cinematic *trompe-l'oeils*, and they have the effect of dragging the spectator out of their detachment and into the story-world of the film.[16]

In practice if not in theory, the two schools of thought can happily coexist, and most films contain a mixture of the two editing styles. Indeed, the point of view cut is really just a variation of Kuleshov.

The third subdivision in the language of film is the most exotic-sounding – *mise en scène*. This is a French term that literally means 'put on to the stage', but which actually refers to everything that is included in the image on screen. Thus lighting, scenery, props, make-up and even the actors' performances all fall within its domain.

The fourth subdivision is sound. This can either be diegetic, when it originates from the film's story-world (e.g dialogue); or non-diegetic, when its source is elsewhere (e.g. the swelling strings that we hear during a love scene).

Let us bring all of these subdivisions together – in particular the first three, which are exclusively visual – by considering a couple of minutes from one

---

16 By a nice coincidence, film theorists have borrowed a term from medicine to describe this process – they speak of 'suturing the viewer into the action.'

of our doctor movies, *The Doctor* (Haines, 1991).[17] (When we watch films, we are usually tied closely to the dialogue. By the simple expedient of pressing the 'mute' button on the remote control, we can allow the visual to rise to pre-eminence.)

This film is about Jack McKee, a surgeon who discovers that he has throat cancer and in consequence rethinks his approach to both his professional and personal life. Our extract begins around eight minutes into the film, by which time we have got to know something of McKee's personality and the work he does; and that he has a ticklish cough.

1.1 [exterior; very long shot + pan] *McKee drives out of the hospital car park in his silver Mercedes convertible, the camera panning with him. The film has been set inside the hospital so far, and now we can see that the building is situated in the heart of downtown in a contemporary American city. As the pan stops, the centre of the frame is occupied by the windscreen of a parked car in which we see the reflection of tall, modern buildings. McKee's car exits the frame left and an ambulance enters it from the right. A silver sign saying 'Hillman Medical Center' can be seen in the background above a doorway through which people in white coats are coming and going. Some trees are visible on the pavement, but they are small and more or less leafless, and surrounded by frames to protect them from the urban bustle.* [This is McKee's high-urgency, up-to-the-minute, acute hospital habitat.]

1.2 [exterior; very long shot] *McKee's journey is not shown in real time (ellipsis is employed) – the Mercedes is now driving up a hill in a residential part of town that has old buildings of only two or three storeys. In the background we see the sky-scraping city centre in its geographic basin below.* [McKee is coming up and out of one world and entering another.]

1.3 [exterior; very long shot + pan] *A pan follows McKee's car as it pulls up in front of a house, the city centre no longer being visible. It is the only flashy car among those parked nearby. The house – like those around it – is constructed partly of wood, and is presentable without being smart. It is on a human scale, and still has its electricity or perhaps phone lines supplied by wires running*

---

17 I would encourage you to hire or buy the movie on DVD and conduct this exercise yourself, perhaps with a friend or colleague. However, the written text will stand on its own.

from wooden poles in the street. Compared with the hospital and city centre, it is middle-class and individual, as opposed to business class and impersonal. The trees on the street are autumnal but healthily so, retaining their rich-coloured foliage; and a creeper is growing up the side of the house. [This other world lives according to different values.]

1.4 [interior; medium close-up] *(Another use of ellipsis – the shot begins in mid-medical examination.) A 45° shot over McKee's right shoulder. An older doctor is using a hand-held torch and spatula to examine McKee's throat. The two men have removed their jackets, and their clothes, although both professional, are markedly different. McKee's shirt is a crisp, striped affair and he is wearing power braces of colours that make no attempt to harmonise; the older doctor, who is his GP, is wearing a waistcoat and floral tie, while the stripes on his shirt are soft to the point of near-invisibility. Behind the men there is a large window. The blinds are down but the slats are half-open, and outside the window we can make out the branches and leaves of a tree.* [This doctor's practice is professional but relatively informal, and not completely divorced from nature.]

1.5 [close-up] *McKee's face over the GP's shoulder. Both men are evidently relaxed, smiling at one another, and at ease with their physical proximity. McKee's face is not brightly lit; indeed, the consulting room as a whole is not brightly lit, with only a chrome standing lamp next to McKee's left shoulder providing artificial light, apart from the examining torch. The room is dappled with natural shadows from the sun filtering through the blinds. Occasionally lights flicker on the wall behind McKee's shoulder – these seem to be reflections from passing cars, because they move quickly and then disappear. So while the blinds preserve confidentiality, they do not shut out the world completely.* [This compromise solution seems to be an objective correlative of the GP's philosophy.]

The usual procedure in this standard way of filming a conversation (called 'shot-countershot') is to film the face of each person in turn as they talk to one another. However, as we hear the GP give his initial assessment (which is provisional but reassuring), the camera remains on McKee's face. This allows us to observe his reaction, which is pensive and largely inscrutable, although his expression(s) suggest that mixed thoughts seem to be passing through his mind. The GP comes back into the frame and feels (palpates) the glands under McKee's jaw. [McKee is not in touch with his feelings, and appears to be afraid to be.]

1.6 [medium close-up + pan] (back to shot 1.4) *The GP's face. The camera pans to follow him walking back to his desk, which is in an adjoining office. His desk, like most of his consulting rooms, is made of old polished wood, confer-ring a natural warmth on the setting. Framed old photographs and diplomas covering the walls add to this, as does the assortment of antique and/or mildly exotic bric-a-brac on the sideboards.* [The set and props reflect the aged-in-the-wood wisdom of the GP.]

1.7 [medium long shot + pan] *The camera is now located in the GP's office; and, in a beautiful composition of horizontals and verticals, McKee is framed by the connecting doorway. There is a pan as McKee collects his jacket and pauses in the doorway itself.* [McKee is elegant but isolated, boxed in by his external surroundings and his internal inhibitions.]

1.8 [medium long shot] *The GP sits in his leather chair writing a prescription. His desk is slightly cluttered, and there is an old-fashioned telephone on it, and a microscope. The bookcase behind him is filled with leather-bound volumes.* [There is something slow-paced and personal about handwriting a prescrip-tion (even though this film was made before computers were as ubiquitous as now!).]

1.9 [medium shot + pan] *McKee, again registering confusing, perhaps con-fused, facial expressions. A pan follows him as he comes from the doorway to stand in front of the GP's desk.* [McKee is struggling with his unacknowl-edged emotions.]

1.10 [medium shot] (back to shot 1.8) *The GP finishes the prescription. He writes with a fountain pen, wears a traditional watch with a leather strap, and has a simple gold wedding ring.* [More and more messages are conveyed that an 'old-fashioned'/traditional doctoring style is 'good.']

1.11 [medium close-up] (back to shot 1.9) *McKee's face appears mildly per-turbed, as if concealing half-felt troubled thoughts.* [McKee is still wrestling with his unexpressed anxieties, and losing.]

1.12 [medium shot] (back to shot 1.10) *The GP hands McKee the prescription.* [The yin-yang ping-pong continues.]

1.13 [medium close-up] (back to shot 1.11) *McKee thanks the GP and reaches forward to shake his hand.* [McKee is gradually reclaiming his accustomed position of being in control.]

1.14 [medium shot] (back to shot 1.12) *The GP extends his right hand, clasps McKee's hand with his left, then holds and shakes McKee's hand affectionately. Both the men's faces are dimly lit, but their hands and forearms come under the table lamplight as they reach towards one another and make contact. McKee's dark, formal suit contrasts with the rolled-up shirt-sleeves of the GP.* [It is perhaps surprising that the GP does not stand up to say good-bye. Perhaps he is allowing McKee to resurrect his self-belief by occupying the more powerful (physical) position in the exchange.]

1.15 [medium shot] (back to shot 1.13) *McKee backs out towards the hallway of the GP's house-cum-surgery, blowing on the freshly inked prescription with what may or may not be fake nonchalance.* [McKee's confident front has been rebuilt.]

The scene has lasted for 1 minute 40 seconds, business having been conducted at a leisurely pace. It is immediately followed by a second consultation, this time conducted by McKee with one of his own patients.

2.1 [interior; medium shot – low angle] *A female patient perches on an examination couch in a hospital, clutching a surgical gown around her, waiting. Her hair is a little unkempt, and her eyes are slightly puffy. Her demeanour indicates upset and anxiety. There is medical equipment attached to the wall, and a lightbox with (what one takes to be) her X-rays in it behind her, as if the shot is giving us a double image of her. A nurse (seen from waist to neck) walks into the frame, puts some equipment down on a table in readiness for the doctor's arrival, and then exits the frame.*

The colours in the room (walls, clothing, and so on) are almost entirely made up of whites and light blues. The nurse's skin is black, which adds visually to the sense of the patient's isolation. Visible surfaces seem flat and two-dimensional. The consulting room is modern and soulless, and offers no comfort to any of its occupants. [The misery of (certain kinds of) patienthood is forcefully conveyed without any dialogue, not least through the setting in which it is played out.]

2.2 [medium close-up + pan] *The door into the room, opening. McKee hurries in. The door is flat and textureless, and is a non-descript shade of black. It has a thin steel frame. Under his white coat, McKee is wearing the same shirt and tie as in the previous scene, the implication being that he has come from his own consultation to this one. The institutional 'uniforms' that all protagonists wear in this scene (unlike the last) serve to depersonalise them. McKee collects the patient's notes from a perspex file holder on the wall next to the door. The camera pans to follow him as he walks briskly past the X-ray images, reading the notes all the while. He looks at the patient's face briefly as he goes past her towards the trolleys where his paraphernalia is laid out, but she is looking downwards. He puts the file down as he finishes studying the notes, and turns back towards the patient, looking directly at her chest. A slight nod of his head indicates that he wants her to open her gown so that he can examine her.* [McKee's consulting style is very different to that of the GP in the previous scene – he is cold and self-absorbed, whereas the other man was warm and interactive.]

2.3 [medium close-up] *The patient seen over McKee's shoulder. A phone – black and box-like, its cord twisted – is visible on the wall over her shoulder. McKee's head and shoulder are in the frame as he moves the patient's gown off her shoulders and looks intently at a surgical scar stretching down the centre of her rib-cage and touches it. Her eyes are turned downwards and sideways, even closed sometimes, as she struggles with her sense of embarrassment and unease. McKee turns away from her and moves out of the frame. As he does so, the X-rays illuminated on the wall behind her are seen more fully. She is left bare-breasted, although the framing softens the awkwardness for the audience, as only the top half of her breasts are in shot. She lifts her eyes to look at McKee.*

[This last shot and the actions in it echo shot 1.7 in the preceding scene. Experientially, this further prompts the viewer to compare scenes that have evidently been put one after the other for that purpose. One difference is that, unlike his GP, McKee doesn't come back into the frame with his patient.]

2.4 [medium shot] *An over-the shoulder shot from behind the patient, as per the shot-countershot practice mentioned earlier. However, in breach of the filmic code, McKee's back is turned. He is washing his hands – good hygiene practice of course, but an action that emphasises his emotional sterility. There is a mirror above the basin, and he glances at the patient in it momentarily before starting to turn and face her. In the event, he only half turns, looking again at the notes while drying his hands and listening to her.* [With the medical agenda of the consultation over, McKee has an opportunity to give some attention to the woman patient herself rather than her operation site; but he fails to take it.]

2.5 [medium close-up] (back to shot 2.3) *The patient smiles a little shyly (while explaining a particular difficulty she is having).* [Again, this echoes McKee-as-patient in shot 1.15, when he was tentatively expressing some anxieties about which he felt embarrassed.]

2.6 [medium shot + pan] (back to shot 2.4) *McKee looks at her face on – the first eye contact that he has made. His eyes are screwed up and his mouth is firmly shut, apparently indicating disapproval or disdain. There is a pan as he moves to his right, taking the patient out of shot. His expressions continue to exude a slightly superior bemusement (an inverted version of his emotionally disconnected facial reactions in the previous scene). Behind him, there are some grey-black blinds (their colour matches the door) covering a narrow window. They are shut so tightly as to make it impossible to know whether any natural light lies behind them.* [Note the contrast with the previous scene.]

2.7 [medium close-up] (back to shot 2.5) *The patient continues to look at, and to, McKee in hope.*

2.8 [medium shot] (back to shot 2.6) *McKee has lost eye contact again while he rearranges his equipment. He re-establishes it momentarily and smiles, more at the ill-judged witticism that he offers than at the patient herself.* [There are two structural comparisons built into this scene – one between McKee and the GP, and the other between McKee and the patient. McKee-as-doctor resembles McKee-as-patient – neither admits the existence of the psyche. Both the GP and the patient seek to make emotional contact with McKee, but he hides behind banter on both occasions.]

2.9 [medium close-up] (back to shot 2.7) *The patient's eyes move away from McKee's face and downwards. She appears resigned to not getting what she wants from him.* [The end of the scene finds the patient in the same place as she was at the start – isolated and unhappy.]

This scene takes place in real time (i.e. there are no ellipses), and lasts for just under a minute. As such, it both feels and is a shorter exchange than that between McKee and his GP; and this is at least partly because McKee as doctor has no time for what he might consider niceties (but what the patient might consider necessities).

For the sake of brevity, and to allow readers to make their own discoveries, I have not included all of the detail I might have added in this cinematic textual analysis (or my running commentary at the end of each shot description). Nonetheless, I hope that it conveys a good deal of what is happening in these two consecutive scenes, and how one might approach their interpretation. There seem to be points made about the way that modern medicine is losing touch with the people it serves even as it makes impressive technical strides; about how the architecture of large institutions can dehumanise the consultation; about how a doctor who is unconnected with his own emotions may be unable to offer support to patients who are experiencing emotional turbulence; and so on. I have deliberately suppressed almost all reference to dialogue in order to illustrate how much of the meaning is contained in images[18] and their juxtaposition.[19]

Earlier in this chapter I mentioned the first coincidence of interests between film and medicine, namely that they both lean heavily on the visual. (In the scenes analysed, there are several instances of medical visuality – for example, the throat examination by the GP, and the X-rays illuminated behind the female patient.) Isolating and studying the visual element of films is a fairly obligatory exercise for anyone who wants to acquire any kind of depth of understanding about how cinema works. And just as the deconstruction of cinematic visuality is helpful in film studies, so the deconstruction of the human body into a series of images is invaluable in the practice of medicine.

---

18 There is of course key non-visual information in the scenes that adds to their resonance – the dialogue is perceptive and affecting in both consultations.

19 The editing of shots is in the 'continuity-editing' style; but the sequence of scenes, and their content, has something of the spirit of Russian montage.

However, the second coincidence is that both film and medicine, generally speaking, have an overriding interest in narrative.[20] We have examined the shots and editing and *mise en scène* in scenes from *The Doctor* in order to better understand the film's story (the choice of McKee's car tells us something about his character; the position of protagonists in the frame tells us something about the power relationships between them; and so on). So, too, should it be in medicine. Images of sickness ought not to be evaluated in isolation from the person from whom they are obtained. It has become almost a clichéd criticism of medical practice that it concentrates on the disease at the expense of the patient – an individual becomes 'an epileptic' rather than 'a person with epilepsy.' (This semantic distinction would be petty and pedantic were it not for the fact that it frequently seems to be indicative of a very real and deep-seated problem.) McKee himself embodies this separation of mind from heart and soul; and the film is a salutary tale about his realisation of this (its source novel was called *A Taste of My Own Medicine*). And the process of studying films, if carried out wisely, can be an experiential way of learning how to separate and then reintegrate. So do try this at home . . .

References

Cartwright L. *Screening the Body: tracing medicine's visual culture*. Minneapolis, MN: University of Minnesota Press; 1995.

Filmography

THE DOCTOR (1991)

Credits

Director	Randa Haines
Producer	Laura Ziskin
Production Company	Touchstone
Screenplay	Robert Caswell
Original story	Ed Rosenbaum
Photography	John Seale

---

20 Not all medicine is interested in narrative, of course (for example, there are branches of research that have little or no patient contact); nor is all cinema narrative-focused (for example, the image-oriented work of the Surrealist film-makers, or the so-called counter-cinema movement of the 1960s). Indeed, only a slab of concrete-reinforced asbestos would deny the huge sensual and aesthetic pleasure there is to be had from movie images in and of themselves. However, for the most part, films are made to tell stories rather than to create beautiful images for their own sake.

Editor	Lisa Fruchtman
Art Director	Ken Adam
Music	Michael Convertino

Cast

Dr Jack McKee	William Hurt
Anne McKee	Christine Lahti
June Ellis	Elizabeth Perkins
Dr Murray Kaplan	Mandy Patinkin
Dr Eli Blumfield	Adam Arkin
Dr Lesley Abbott	Wendy Crewson

CHAPTER 6

Deep and meaningful:
Le Corbeau

In the last chapter we looked at one way of working out what films mean – the practice of textual analysis. There are others; because although the close scrutiny of scenes provides raw data, it does not provide context.

The Raven is a film with an unusual storyline: a doctor who is new to a small town is the subject of a poison pen letter condemning his embryonic but unconsummated affair with the blonde wife of a colleague. A string of letters to other townspeople follow, all of which touch on sore points of the recipients. Soon the town is awash with suspicion and mutual accusation. Senior local figures propose various means of putting a stop to the letters; and several are tried without success. As the atmosphere becomes increasingly rancorous, the doctor starts an affair with a different woman, a club-footed brunette with hypochondriacal tendencies and a bad reputation. One of the hospital patients commits suicide; one of the hospital nurses is hounded and then (wrongly) arrested for writing the letters; a child attempts suicide on discovering via a letter that she is not biologically related to her father. Another doctor – the cuckolded colleague – admits to an addiction to morphine, which a former lover (the incarcerated hospital nurse) has been stealing for him from hospital. The brunette throws herself down the stairs in an attempt to terminate her pregnancy by the doctor/lover, who himself is suspected of performing illegal abortions. The troubles are finally brought to an end when the cuckold's wife is (wrongly) committed to a mental institution, and the mystery letter-writer is murdered by the mother of the suicide victim. The film has a convoluted storyline, to put it mildly, and sometimes it is hard to verify its chain of cause and effect; but the viewer is swept along from one dramatic scene to another.

Ponder for a moment what you would say, on the basis of the above account, if you were asked where and when you thought this film had been made and what it was about.

How might you modify your answer if you were told that it was made in France in 1943? You would no doubt wonder if the film was related to the Second World War in some way. And on further reflection, you might replace the 'if' with 'how'; because, directly or indirectly, a film is a reflection of its time. Perhaps you know already that occupying German forces encouraged the writing of anonymous letters as a way of rooting out Jews and members of the Resistance. The film is set in a non-specific although contemporary time period, and no mention is made of the war, but the parallel is what the French call *incontournable* (un-get-roundable!).[21] However, let us be a little more systematic in our speculations, because *Le Corbeau* (to give its French title) is a complex artefact, and it repays prolonged attention.

With regard to the film's background, it was based (as the phrase goes) on a true story, there having been an outbreak of poison pen letters in the 1920s in Tulle, a small provincial town in southern France. One could easily envisage it as a melodrama, but in fact it is constructed as a mystery-thriller of sorts – that is, the film's events are driven by the advent of the letters; and the film ends when the poison penman is identified and justice is dispensed. However, that conventional framework carries unusual baggage, as we have seen. Film-making, like many walks of French life during the Occupation, was fraught with difficulties of both a moral and practical nature. Much of the cinematic establishment had headed for the (Beverly) hills in the face of war, which created openings for others, the only problem being that the newcomers' artistic hands were tightly tied by political cords.[22] *Le Corbeau* was made by one such director, the relatively inexperienced Henri-Georges Clouzot, under the auspices of Continental Films, a production company set up in Paris by Goebbels to turn out lightweight cinematic fare (as opposed to overt propaganda) as a diversion for the public. As such, *Le Corbeau* was both a great success and a serious failure – as befits such a protean film! – because it was very popular with cinema-goers (i.e. it was a commercial hit)

---

21 The initial intertitle reads 'Une petite ville, ici ou ailleurs', and the second phrase is mistranslated in the subtitle as 'anywhere', rather than 'here or elsewhere', which is much more pointed.

22 For a fascinating cinematic depiction of the situation, watch *Laissez-Passer* (Tavernier, 2001).

and very unpopular with just about everyone else. The public seem to have responded to its substance as if they were at last getting a decent meal after being kept on a diet of *amuse-gueules*.[23] However, the authorities took a dimmer view. The Church saw it as blasphemous, because of various scenes in which solemn religious rites were undercut – usually by black humour, not to say mockery; the Vichy government (which was in charge of unoccupied but German-controlled France) tried to block the film's distribution because they felt that it portrayed the very aspects of French national identity that needed to be extirpated if France was ever to rebuild itself; the Gestapo didn't like the film because its central theme, so *they* felt, was a critique of anonymous denunciation – the very activity that they were seeking to encourage in the local population. Even the would-be Free French (hidden among the populace) condemned it, because they felt that it showed French character in such an appalling light that it was effectively aiding and abetting the enemy. Certainly, if films were graded according to the quantity of debate that they generated, *Le Corbeau* was an instant masterpiece!

The upshot of all this was that Clouzot was debarred from further work in the cinema (a ban that was only lifted two years after the war ended), and the film was withdrawn from circulation. (It reached an expectant England in 1948 and garnered mixed reviews. Some critics found it distasteful, while others considered it to be incisive.)

Thus the reception of *Le Corbeau* does not allow us to reach any conclusion about what its 'message' might be. On the contrary, we are confronted by the apparent contradiction that it was denounced by parties (the collaborating French, the non-collaborating French, and the occupying Germans) who ought not to have shared opinions on anything.

If we turn to more academic approaches, we continue to find divergent views, although perhaps with a little less mutual exclusivity. The film historian would argue that *Le Corbeau* was a notable forerunner of American 'film noir.' Certainly the film has many of the qualities that would later come to be associated with that genre, both in its themes – which everyone seems to agree represent a bleak view of humanity – and in its cinematography, which creates striking images of shadows and light, thus evoking the contrast between good and bad which is central to the narrative. (In one scene, Vorzet, the cuckolded older doctor, and Germain, the doctor who is the notional central character, are discussing good and evil in a night-darkened room. Vorzet swings the

---

23 Appetisers that accompany pre-dinner drinks.

bright, naked bulb hanging from the ceiling to indicate how light and dark are movable rather than fixed areas.)

The film scholar who is interested in gender issues also finds much of interest in the film. Male characters initially occupy all the positions of power – both formally and informally – and yet prove to be power*less* to stem the tide of letters and their problematic consequences. There are several scenes in which high-ranking men in the town debate what steps to take, but all the courses of action prove equally ineffectual. (The most amusing of these is a marathon enforced dictation in the school classroom to which (adult) suspects are collectively subjected, the idea being to identify the culprit via their handwriting. The texts dictated – much to the shock of those being tested – are the poison pen letters themselves: 'You *débauché*' [repeated slowly], 'You have been playing around with the wife of . . . [repeated slowly] 'You – have – been – playing – around – with –' and so on!) This perceived male inadequacy would have had a special resonance in a country whose men had just lost a war in a blaze of ingloriousness. The sound of deflating masculinity is accompanied, at least in part, by that of women gradually taking control. For instance, the club-footed brunette undergoes something of a physical and moral rehabilitation in the course of the film; and the final retribution is exacted by a cleaning lady, who takes the work of both the police and the judiciary into her own hands in order to see justice done. However, it should be emphasised that the film does not constitute an unmitigated paean to female supremacy. At its denouement, a relatively innocent party – Vorzet's wife – is despatched to a lunatic asylum unwarrantedly; and the female behaviour in the film in general is not notably superior to that of the male characters.

From an ideological viewpoint, the film also seems equivocal. Is it espousing a kind of Nietzschean contempt for the feckless local population as a whole as well as for the individual men (and women) of whom it is comprised, virtually all the protagonists proving to be weak or corrupted? This interpretation would endorse the view that a strong outsider is required to come in and improve things ('Welcome, Herr Hitler!'). Or is it rather a leftist attack on the pusillanimous petits bourgeois who had run France for too long, letting it decline to the point where it was easy prey for its fascist neighbours ('Comrades, rise up!')?

Then there is the auteur angle – the consideration of Clouzot's directorial traits as a clue to the meaning of this particular example of his oeuvre. (In this context it is worth noting that Clouzot also wrote the film, with the help of screenplay writer Louis Chavance.) His two most famous subsequent films were *Le Salaire de la Peur* (*Wages of Fear*) (1953) and *Les Diaboliques* (*Diabolique*) (1955), which were both international hits. The former is the story of four down-on-their-uppers expatriate truck drivers in South America who agree to drive a convoy of nitroglycerine on a highly dangerous mountain route because they are desperate for money and a sense of purpose. The journey becomes a physical and metaphysical descent into hell. *Les Diaboliques* is the story of schoolteachers who plot to kill one of their number, and succeed. The two films share *Le Corbeau*'s dark view of human relationships, a mistrust of those who exercise authority, and X-ray vision for moral fibre fatigue. As a result, Clouzot has sometimes been accused of being an amoral director. However, this judgement is surely inaccurate – those such as Clouzot who dissect morality in order to demonstrate its shortcomings are usually the people who are most concerned about it. Another label that is given to Clouzot is that of 'the French Hitchcock', and (if used in moderation) this is a much better judgement. There are definite similarities between the two men, including their interest in pre-shooting preparation (often storyboarding the entire film in advance) and general perfectionism; their evident relish for exploring the dark side of man; their injection of black humour into cinematic set-pieces (in *Le Corbeau*, a particularly revelatory poison pen letter appears to emanate from the coffin of the suicide victim during the funeral procession through town). Certainly Clouzot has a highly distinctive artistic vision – the kind of powerful identity that makes watching one of his films more like a soak in a scented bath[24] than a quick shower. In the context of his other films, *Le Corbeau* can be seen as fairly typical; and so we might conclude that the particular circumstances of the early 1940s simply enabled him to make this film then, allowing him to work in the cracks between the political paving stones in order to express something very personal and almost timeless. Certainly it seems miraculous now that the film – given its pin-sharp critique of such salient contemporary issues, and the hyper-vigilant control of the authorities at the time – was ever allowed to be made, let alone screened.

Academic critical theories sometimes seem to be vying with one another to reveal the 'true meaning' of a piece of art. However, there is a school of thought that manages to be more inclusive, due to a certain built-in flexibility. This is because it factors in the hitherto overlooked third party in Art's eternal triangle. If first we have the artist and his or her intentions; and secondly the work of art that they create; then thirdly we must have the reader

---

24 In '*Eau des fleurs du mal*', perhaps.

(or spectator, or listener, etc.), taken collectively and individually. From this premise, *Le Corbeau* might not – indeed cannot – have one 'real' meaning. A French audience seeing it in 1943 would experience a different film to a French audience watching it today. And if I watch the film as someone who has a club-foot, or an unfaithful wife, my sympathies – or empathies – may cause my take on the film to differ from yours, as someone who has experienced injustice caused by malicious rumour or whatever. To some extent, then, every member of every audience sees what they want to see and hears what they want to hear when they watch this (or any other) film; and they are entitled to do so. However, to accept this is not to embrace the modus operandi of Speakers' Corner. In the first place, the starting point for all discussion of meanings must be a scrupulously close study of the film itself; and in the second place, there must be a recognition that with any freedom comes responsibility, here taking the form of acknowledging one's interpretive baggage. Our baggage in this book is that of habitual doctor-watchers, and *Le Corbeau* certainly provides grist for our mill.

These medics are a cankered bunch, notwithstanding their socially acceptable appearances and self-assured emanations of respectability. Their words and deeds are no better, and indeed may be slightly worse, than all the other vain and self-preserving 'senior figures' who are running the town's affairs. For instance, they are not distinguished from this cadre by a higher code of ethical behaviour. We first see them in a hospital corridor bickering with one another and opting out of social responsibility. One is a mild alcoholic, unhappily married to 'a virago'; and when he accuses the hospital's bursar of embezzlement, a counter-accusation about his improprieties with the latter's daughter is enough to make him drop the matter. This doctor is also the father of the town's public prosecutor, whose policies he tries to influence by invoking his parental authority.

Meanwhile, doctors occupy two of the three most important roles in the story (the third role being that of the self-reforming brunette Denise). For the majority of the film, the touchstone of sanity and informed thinking is the elderly psychiatrist Vorzet. We first meet him on his return from a trip to a psychiatric conference; and his witty and sceptical commentary about the proceedings is both immediately endearing and credibility-building: 'The only thing more ridiculous than a medical congress is a congress of psychiatrists. Nobody listens to the person who is talking – thank God; because if they did, they would hear an enormous river of rubbish. Only an audience of sick people would take such communications seriously!'

This manner of address – each statement a pronouncement on the way of the world – marks him out from almost everyone else in the town; and accordingly people look to him for guidance at various stages. In fact he continues to claim the moral and intellectual high ground until the film's penultimate shot. Yet our trust in him is reduced to near breaking point – first, by steady depletion, because empirical evidence repeatedly fails to support his contentions (for example, his prescriptions for dealing with the letter-writing are entirely unsuccessful); and secondly, because it turns out that he is 'le corbeau.' This revelation throws retrospective doubt on all of his utterances, of course. Were they as false as his identity?[25] This would be fine for the audience's sense of moral orderliness, and in the great tradition of the surprise-twist whodunnit, if there was some kind of pillar of strength to turn to, a hero on whom we could pin our hopes. However, we only have Dr Germain, the subject of the first letter, and he is a flawed specimen.

We are introduced to Germain in the first scene as he emerges, grim-faced and with blood on his hands, from an unsuccessful home delivery. He is unsympathetic (and certainly unapologetic) about the event, and appears to have an odd attitude to mothers and babies, which leads to the accusations (which are not entirely incredible) that he is an abortionist. Nonetheless, he is apparently the hero of the film. Not only does the story revolve around him, but he is played by Pierre Fresnay, the biggest name[26] in the cast. In the course of the film he sometimes behaves admirably, but frequently displays anti-heroic tendencies. He is selfish and self-righteous in his dealings with women, and vacillates feebly in his relationships with them; he is generally grumpy (even with children); he seems to have not much courage and fewer convictions (except to do what he wants when he wants). The greatest blame that accrues to him is when he is easily persuaded to sign the certificate committing Vorzet's wife (whom he knows well and has been at least partially in love with) to a mental asylum. It is a deeply unsettling scene when she is carted away in the ambulance, physically resisting and protesting her innocence all the while. (It turns out that she is innocent, but the miscarriage of justice remains uncorrected.) This unappetising cake is glazed by Denise's evaluations of him during their verbal duels: 'You're cowardly, you're weak.

---

25 It is noteworthy, and very much in the spirit of the film, that the credibility of at least his philosophical observations is actually not compromised by his ultimate guilt.

26 It is painful for the fans he made via his participation in Renoir's sublime *La Grande Illusion* to see him in the compromised surroundings of a Continental film.

You'll always remain the saddest of creatures!' 'A fool?' 'No – a bourgeois!' To which response Germain offers no rebuttals. On the positive side, he is intellectually robust and no pushover in social intercourse; and his backstory, which is revealed late in the film, does go some way towards explaining his behaviour (although it does not excuse it). And by the end he has turned into someone who has abandoned his attempts to preserve neutrality (he claims that he wants 'neither friends nor enemies') in favour of a reawakened ability to love. However, this chink of optimistic light in an otherwise very dark room is arguably the least believable aspect of the film. Perhaps Clouzot felt obliged to allow some degree of happy ending. Or possibly it was part of the director's master plan, because paradoxically it precipitates Germain's first clinical mistake – the consigning of his former paramour to an asylum. What price personal happiness?! So while we might want to side with Germain, and indeed often do so in the face of unjust accusations, he is no knight on a white charger, either medical or moral. It is perhaps the combination of his shortcomings as a conventional hero and Vorzet's as a conventional villain (i.e. he is arguably the wisest character in the film) that embodies one of the film's most important messages, which is both timeless and also absolutely pertinent to France in 1943. It is summed up in Vorzet's words to Germain under the swinging light bulb: 'When I look in the mirror, I see a devil and an angel. You think that people are all good or all bad. You think that good is light and darkness is evil. But where is the shade? Where is the light? Where is the frontier of evil? Do you know which side of it you're on? When people are pushed, they do bad things; and you would too.' By the end of the film, Germain has reluctantly accepted this: 'It's a terrible thing to say, but evil is necessary. It's like an illness from which you recover strengthened.' That's a hard pill to swallow even now, let alone in the middle of World War Two.

Is this, then, what *Le Corbeau* really 'means'? Well – definitely, maybe . . .

Acknowledgement

I am very grateful to Lydia Collingridge, Rory Conn and Nick Hulme for their enthusiastic and efficient help with the preparation of this chapter.

Further reading

Ehrlich E. French film during the German Occupation: the case of *Le Corbeau*. *Wide Angle*. 1981; **4**: 12–17.

Mayne J. *Le Corbeau*. French Film Guides Series. Urbana, IL: University of Illinois Press; 2007.

The UK DVD release of the film (produced in 2005 by Optimum Home Entertainment) has a very informative commentary by Ginette Vincendeau.

Filmography

LE CORBEAU (1943)

Credits

Director	Henri-Georges Clouzot
Producer	Réné Montis
Production Company	Continental Films
Scenario	Louis Chavance
Screenplay	Henri-Georges Clouzot, Louis Chavance
Photography	Nicolas Hayer
Editor	Marguerite Beaugé
Art Director	Andrei Andrejew
Music	Tony Aubin

Cast

Dr Rémy Germain	Pierre Fresnay
Denise Saillens	Ginette Leclerc
Laura Vorzet	Micheline Francey
Dr Vorzet	Pierre Larquey
Marie Corbin	Hélèna Manson
Cancer victim's mother	Sylvie
Haberdasher	Jeanne Fusier-Gir

CHAPTER 7

Wars of the world

The film described in the previous chapter was made during a war, but was not (at least overtly) about that war. The films in this chapter all have war at their centre, but were all (with one exception) products of peacetime. It is perhaps tautological to note that a nation can only reflect on its wars retrospectively, as it is too busy fighting for its life at the time of them, a situation that demands unequivocal and unhesitating patriotism, not doubts or criticisms.

A Matter of Life and Death (Powell and Pressburger, 1946)

This film has a wonderful beginning, and its middle and end are not bad either. English pilot Peter Carter is returning from a bombing raid over Germany in 1945. His plane is in flames and unlandable; his crew have baled out on his orders, but his own parachute has been shot to ribbons. He is planning to jump to his death (in preference to burning alive), and we see him do this. However, before he does so, he is contacted by base; and he strikes up a conversation with the radio operator, with whom he shares his last thoughts. Of course the radio operator is a woman; and of course they fall in love in the space of two minutes. Notwithstanding this cheap-point sentimental element, there is an irresistible poignancy to their dialogue, spoken as it is through stiff upper lips. And this is no clichéd version of British heroism: the woman is American, for a start; and Carter is a bright young poet who quotes Marvell and Raleigh and is bubbling over with expressivity. Accordingly, their fast-forward romance seems far from implausible. Then a magical thing happens (and 'magical' is not a word that one associates with British war films). Carter is washed up on the English coast, a little battered but certainly unbowed; and he immediately meets and instantly recognises the radio operator, cycling home from her night duty; and their affair picks up where it left off a few hours before. It turns out that the conductor allocated to spirit the pilot to heaven missed him in the night-time fog, and that there is hell to pay as a result of the celestial books being unbalanced at close of play. The film, as its title makes clear, is about Carter trying to hang on to his place in the real world when his presence is required in the hereafter.

However, Carter is only half the hero of the film. The audience wants him to stay alive and keep the girl of course; but he is a more or less passive participant, his activities being largely confined to recuperative sleep, parrying the verbal thrusts of the heavenly conductor trying to lure him upwards, or exchanging professions of love with his girlfriend. In fact, at the climax of the film he is under ether! The more important protagonist – in terms both of character and of steering the film's narrative – is Dr Frank Reeves. Here is an incarnation of the kind of man on whom post-war Britain was evidently pinning its hopes. Adjectives such as 'modest', 'brilliant', 'well read', 'open-minded', 'sympathetic', 'proactive', 'kindly' and 'selfless'[27] are drawn to him in the course of the film like iron filings to a magnet. He is the doctor in the village near the RAF base where June (the radio operator) takes Peter. However, it quickly becomes apparent that he is no 'mere' village doctor. June nails this early on, despite Reeves' attempts to downplay himself:

> June: 'You're only a village doctor because you like to live in a village. Dr McEwen says that what you don't know about neurology would fit inside a peanut.'
>
> Reeves: 'Oh – I'm a good guesser . . .'

Not only has he observed rare brain operations at the Hôpital de la Pitié in Paris, but he knows his English culture inside out. Indeed, one feels that it is his acquaintance with the metaphysical poets that allows him to understand Carter's case. He not only detects sense in the pilot's apparently deranged accounts of heaven-sent emissaries and death forestalled, but he also recognises the all-conquering power of love. Far from dismissing the pilot's strange tale, he embraces it, emphasising that Carter must win his trial in heaven (he

---

27 Of which 'sexless' is a subset. One gets the impression that he is a bachelor because being a good husband would draw him away unforgivably from his duty, which is to make people better.

has been granted a hearing) if he is to survive on earth. At the same time, he is closely observing Carter to work out the precise location in his brain where an operation is needed in order to save his life medically. The climax of the film is its trial scene. Reeves has died (thanks to his proclivity for tearing along country lanes on his motorcycle) just in time to act as Carter's defending counsel – the only representative whom Carter feels happy with, notwithstanding his right to choose any (dead) person in history! Inevitably, Reeves gets to say some important lines at this point that express the ideals underpinning the film. The hard-fought ethical–legal battle is played out in heaven at the same time as Carter is undergoing his critical brain operation on earth at the hands of skilled surgeons. The parallel and interlinked worlds of the physical and the metaphysical have rarely been so adroitly woven together, making *A Matter of Life and Death* virtually a manifesto for the discipline of medical humanities. It is also one of the great works of British cinema, its atypicality being rooted in its joint creators, the immensely imaginative and intellectually advanced Michael Powell and Emeric Pressburger (a cinematic double act being atypical in itself).

Before we move on, there is another aspect of the film that is worth noting. While the majority of it seems as fresh as ever today, this other element shows signs of age. When we first meet the doctor, he is up in his darkened study projecting images of the village – obtained through a home-made camera obscura – on to a white garden table. Rather like a submariner with a periscope, he scours the locality, commentating to himself as he does ('There goes old Mary, looking quite skittish . . .').[28] June breaks in on him and remarks 'Surveying your kingdom?'; to which Reeves replies, 'The village doctor has to know everything. You'd be surprised by how many diagnoses I've formed up here.' Michel Foucault would have had a fit. Later, when June introduces him to Peter in the recreation room of the manor house that has been billeted for troops, Reeves asks a series of diagnostic questions. On the one hand, there is nothing exceptional in this, and yet, perhaps because of the non-medical setting, the exchange seems extraordinary now. Reeves only asks questions, and he gives no answers (perhaps because no one asks him for any). He is plainly formulating a diagnosis, but neither the cinema audience, the patient nor the patient's carer (June) is party to even a hint of what it might be. And no one (in the film) thinks that this is strange! In fact, when a little later on

---

28 The medical humanities link is made pretty explicitly at this point, too, when Reeves talks about seeing the whole town 'all together, as in a poet's eye.'

he does start to share some clinical information about Peter with June, he quickly pulls himself up (apparently to spare her the gory details), saying 'I'm not going to tell you any more.' And what is her response? 'Thanks!' Plainly, this was a time when benevolent paternalism was fine by all; and as we have seen, the whole story is predicated on the trust vested in a member of the medical profession. We may not feel so sanguine about the terms of this social contract today. Yet some of us might admit to having a few recidivist cells that react involuntarily and generate a twinge of envy of apparently simpler times.

Dive Bomber (Curtiz, 1941)

A film that stars Errol Flynn and has the title *Dive Bomber* would seem a safe bet for 90 minutes of action and excitement. Yet it is quite easy to nod off for the odd ten minutes during its two-hour-plus running time, and if you do so, you won't miss much. However, although most people will find *Dive Bomber* dull, it is a field day for the film buff (and, incidentally, for the plane-spotter); and if you have got this far in this book you either already are, or are well on the way to becoming, a film buff.

In North American terms, the film was made just before World War Two – that is to say, production took place during the early months of 1941 and it was released that August. (The Japanese attacked Pearl Harbor on 7 December of the same year, precipitating America's participation in the war.) The film has a doctor as its hero, but he is an odd kind of doctor and an odd kind of hero.

Errol Flynn was the cinematic swashbuckler par excellence, who seemed happy to stay in role in his private life, at least to judge by his appetite for alcohol and women (a trait which only added to his box-office appeal). The phrase 'in like Flynn' may even have been invented in honour of his wicked ways, although there is some uncertainty about this. He was probably the biggest action hero of the late 1930s, the go-to guy if you wanted to get some undiluted virility up on the screen. So it is somewhat disconcerting to watch him in *Dive Bomber* apparently systematically dismantling this persona and replacing it with something far more muted and appropriate to the prevailing political circumstances. It seems that, on this occasion at least, Hollywood was as sensitive a weather vane about the imminence of war as any diplomatic communiqués.

Flynn is already on the road to reconstruction when the film starts. He is a doctor assigned to the US armed forces rather than an adventurer of some sort.[29] (Moreover, he goes further down that road when he submits himself to retraining as a specialist.) This immediately signals his shift from the physical to the mental plane. The plot, such as it is, centres on the efforts of flight surgeons and pilots to resolve the problem of variable atmospheric pressure in small aircraft, and its debilitating effects on pilots. There is plenty of aerial photography, with stunning images, beautifully filmed by our old friend Bert Glennon (*see* Chapter 3), which seem to be there for their own sake (insofar as they do not further the story at all). These surely constitute the subliminal part of the message that flying a war-plane is something worth doing. There are many test flights, and these episodes supply the film's only tension (manufactured though it is), effectively constituting a rehearsal for the real deal that is on the horizon. A fair amount of prosaic research takes place in laboratories, these scenes conveying the message that the military is being mindful to harness the best that science can offer. There is little doubt that all this is gearing the nation for World War Two, as allusions are made to troubles elsewhere in the world, and to the likelihood of US involvement sooner or later. As previously noted, the film's title is something of a con, promising more action than it delivers. Certainly it is an unnecessarily long movie. Is it deliberately slowing down the pace to confound expectations and thereby make the audience stop and think? It is certainly tempting to accept this interpretation in hindsight.

Running alongside the thin storyline is the interesting stuff concerning Flynn's makeover. At the beginning he is something of an individualist. A self-assured 'Harvard, Hopkins and Cambridge man', he bridles at figures of authority, and can be brusque in his dealings with less exalted folk. The film charts his journey to enlightenment in the form of recognition of the contribution of others, and of the necessity of teamwork in the face of complex problems. He does not perform any life-saving heroics as a flight surgeon (indeed he is helpless to save people on more than one occasion), instead committing himself to one-step-at-a-time research into means of primary prevention. At the same time, we see the complete deactivation of his sexuality, as he is pursued by women whom he absent-mindedly spurns because he is preoccupied with his work. (In one memorable scene, he and a colleague end

---

29 He was also a doctor at the start of *Captain Blood* (Curtiz, 1935), the movie that made his name. However, in that film he metamorphosed into a pirate captain, whence his image never looked back, thus making it some kind of sibling to *Dive Bomber*.

up wrecking a cosy two-couple dinner date by getting carried away drawing scientific diagrams on the restaurant tablecloth.) We also see his two-fisted ruggedness put back in the box. There is a trivial road-rage punch-up (presumably because a Flynn film without a fight would be a breach of the Trade Descriptions Act) that soon ends up with him apologising to his opponent and helping him to his feet. This is hardly the stuff of Robin Hood versus Guy of Gisborne.[30] And we see him hand on the very mantle of hero to his two closest collaborators, who are determinedly 'ordinary' (insofar as they are played by unglamorous actors and have no self-regard). The last scene takes place on a parade ground, with Flynn merging almost completely into the uniformed group. The three men have had to work hard at accepting each other, their initial discord being only gradually superseded by harmony born out of mutual respect. The accommodation of differences, and the price (in terms of self-sacrifice) of progress, are both constant themes of the film. So *Dive Bomber* might have been called '*The Emasculation of Errol*', or perhaps a more overarching title would be '*The Maturation of Malehood.*' As such, it manages to be a pro-war film that is entirely non-bellicose.

Regeneration (Mackinnon, 1997)

The patron saint of anti-war films – as indeed it may be of anti-war novels – is *All Quiet On the Western Front* (Milestone, 1930). However, that film will not detain us, as the doctors in it are merely functionaries who do not own their screen time. One of its honourable descendants is *Regeneration* (which is also drawn from a First World War literary source – Pat Barker's trilogy of the same name).

Real-life doctor William Rivers has in his charge two real-life patients in the shape of Wilfred Owen and Siegfried Sassoon; as well as other, invented patients (notably a working-class officer called Prior). You might expect the story to focus on the famous poets (huge figures in English literature), with emotional mileage being made of Owen's premature death in particular. In fact the narrative takes a far more original approach, and the doctor is crucial to it.

Sassoon is a decorated officer who is liked and respected by his men for his care, consideration and bravery. He is in fact half in love with the war, and a vigorous participant in it, despite his abhorrence of it. Notwithstanding this,

---

30 One of the greatest of all film swordfights-to-the-death, seen in Flynn's *Robin Hood* (Keighley, 1938).

he has written an incisive anti-war declaration (or more accurately, an anti-authorities declaration) that is causing considerable discomfort in political circles, and he is therefore sent to Craiglockhart Hospital in Scotland (where he meets Owen). It is hoped that Rivers, a psychiatrist at the hospital, will pronounce him mad or cure him of the mental 'sickness' that is giving rise to such 'unpatriotic' views. The two men are therefore pitted against each other, even though their natural predispositions might have put them on the same side (and ensure that they like each other). Sassoon can see what a sympathetic and honest figure Rivers is, and how he brings considerable compassion and skill[31] to his job; while Rivers is neither so naive (the date is 1917) nor blindly nationalistic as to believe that the war is being prosecuted for noble reasons and according to sound strategy. So while the film charts the outward fight between the two men to claim the moral and intellectual high ground, at the same time we see each of them struggling with internal battles. For Sassoon, this essentially involves squaring his rejection of the *casus belli* with his sense of solidarity with his fellow soldiers. For Rivers, the dilemma is twofold. First, he realises that he is complicit in sustaining a status quo – the political endorsement of carnage on a vast scale – in which he does not believe; and secondly, he knows that he is 'taking a sane man [Sassoon] and making him mad enough to go back to war.' (The phrase is reminiscent of the notorious *Catch-22*, which was thought up in response to the next world war.)

During the course of the film there is a gradual transfer of what might be described as positivity. Sassoon, who starts off disenchanted and isolated, finds himself drawn ineluctably back to the shared experience of the front. Rivers, who is reasonably confident of his place in the world when we first meet him, slowly crumbles under the barrage of horrific truths to which Sassoon and other war-damaged patients expose him.[32] A turning point comes when Sassoon opts for a compromise course of action in his fight with the authorities because he thinks of Rivers' needs as well as his own. It is a nice

---

31 He is seen to be the most understanding and enlightened doctor (mention is made of his new-fangled Freudian beliefs) in what is already an extremely benevolent institution for its time.

32 As Rivers, actor Jonathan Pryce subtly conveys the fragility of a man who cares too much about people to be able to cope in the midst of an exercise in mass cruelty to humanity. This strand of the film shows how war touched those at home as well as on the front. Rivers' decomposition, which stemmed precisely from his merits, is one of the saddest elements of the film – even sadder in some ways than the death of one of Britain's most famous poets, because at least we know about this in advance.

paradox that Sassoon wins his personal battle (and even survives a sniper's bullet by a hair's breadth having returned to the frontline); while Rivers apparently loses his. The last shot is of Rivers sitting alone in Craiglockhart reading a poem of Owen's that Sassoon has sent him and crying. War damages many, and in many ways.

Doctors have an obvious, almost automatic role in war (and its associated films) because the harm that is done to human bodies and minds when countries take up arms requires expert repair. The task of doctors as an essential adjunct puts them in a special position – they are once removed from the core business of fighting, while being inextricably, intimately and professionally bound up with it. (Thanks to its supposed scientific detachment and consequent relative neutrality, medicine can be a buffer zone, a no-man's-land where only the Red Cross flag flies.) Thus war-film doctors are well placed (in physical and narratological terms) to provide some kind of commentary on events – a point that echoes, in slightly altered form, the one made in the opening paragraph of this chapter. The nature of that commentary is of course determined by circumstance – that is to say, the preoccupations of the given film.[33] So in *A Matter of Life and Death*, Reeves articulately explores what kinds of values were considered worth defending in World War Two, with a view to working out how to rebuild after it. Conversely, Doug Lee (Flynn) in *Dive Bomber* is a palimpsest presenting the processes that a country needs to undergo before a war. These films were made on either side of and within touching distance of World War Two;[34] and their focus is on national identity and its relationship to individuality. *Regeneration* was about a war that had less clear ideological ends; rather, the First World War has become culturally synonymous with a futility bordering on absurdity. The film is interested in the toll that this absurdity takes on individuals, including Rivers. His type of doctoring brings him into close contact with the psyches of his patients, and as a result, the detachment that we alluded to earlier decreases, and the distinction between doctor and patient begins to blur.

---

33 We are focusing on fiction films. Documentaries, such as *Let There Be Light* (Huston, 1945), warrant a separate discussion, and readers are directed to CA Morgan's chapter in the book *Signs of Life: Medicine and Cinema* (Wallflower Press, 2005).

34 World War Two is perhaps rare in that good and evil were unusually clearly delineated. Historians don't like to talk about a 'just war', because of the cultural relativity involved in such a phrase. Nonetheless, the breadth and depth of opprobrium heaped on Nazism make World War Two unusually clear-cut.

MASH (Altman, 1970)

Our last film, *MASH*, is the exception in the chapter, insofar as it was made when the USA was engaged in a war. However, there is an element of leger-demain here, because the war depicted is the Korean War, while the film was made at the time of the Vietnam War – although it is hard to tell the difference when watching.[35] In part it is this deception that allows the film-makers to re-create the critical distance that we have referred to earlier. In part also, though, the film is self-consciously a product of its era – an era in which counter-culture was king (or at least a threat to the throne).

It may also be the last major film in which doctors are unequivocal heroes (although this kind of statement is very vulnerable to contradiction!), and as such represents an important landmark in shifting societal attitudes to medicine. We have been using the term 'hero' fairly loosely to refer to the main protagonist in our doctors-at-war films. However, in *MASH* it takes on the word's additional sense, which is that of representing a positive fantasy of how we might like to be. In this film, many viewers (and not just medical ones) will side enthusiastically with the two main doctors because of their attractive attributes. (There are of course more recent films in which a doctor is heroic, but these tend to be in the thriller genre.) In *MASH*, medicine's two good rep-resentatives – for not all the medics in the film are on a par – are the last line of sanity in a mad world, the practice of medicine being the only decent thing that an individual can do (in contrast, Father Mulcahy, the representative of organised religion, is patently out of his depth). Dr Pierce and Dr McIntyre are not only ultra-hip and witty and technically skilled (and good at American football), but they also demonstrate more social responsibility than anyone else, simultaneously patching up society's casualties and undermining at every possible opportunity the authority figures who are implicated in causing so much trauma. (The contrast with *Catch-22* (Nichols, 1970), another anti-war film made at almost exactly the same time, is striking. Like *MASH*, this film is set in a previous war (World War Two), but here the doctors are weak and unassertive, and so find themselves positioned as 'one of them' rather than 'one of us.') In short, they are role models for a disaffected youth that none-theless does not want to completely renounce its place in society (compared

---

35 You have to look and listen very closely to find anything in the film to indicate that it is *not* the Vietnam War which is being portrayed – an early intertitle, the odd item on the camp tannoy, but not much else. By contrast, hairstyles, dress, attitude, etc. are all emphatically contemporaneous with the production date.

with the two main protagonists in, say, the roughly contemporaneous *Easy Rider* (Hopper, 1969), who are simply alienated). No wonder it is a firm favourite[36] with many doctors.

MASH is the most commercially successful of all of the films described in this chapter, and certainly has the best-known title thanks to the long-running TV series that it spawned. (Are there any readers of this book who do not know that it is a black comedy documenting life in a US field hospital during the Korean War?) Although it takes a ruthlessly bleak view of war – many scenes are spent fairly gruesomely in blood-spattered operating rooms – *MASH* evinces a paradoxical degree of optimism. This stems from both the sense of community that we see being engendered by war (and the practice of medicine); and from the fact that so much of the film is quite simply extremely funny. Curiously, then, it turns out to be a feel-good movie, and so a chapter that has brushed up against Man's most violent and destructive tendencies ends on a tenuously upbeat note.

Further reading

Haslam D. Medical classics: M*A*S*H. *BMJ*. 2007; **334**: 47.

Morgan CA III. From *Let There Be Light* to *Shades of Grey*: the construction of authoritative knowledge about combat fatigue (1945–48). In: Harper G, Moor A (eds) *Signs of Life: medicine and cinema*. London: Wallflower Press; 2005.

Filmography

A MATTER OF LIFE AND DEATH (1946)

Credits

Directors	Michael Powell, Emeric Pressburger
Producers	Michael Powell, Emeric Pressburger
Production Companies	Archers Film Productions, J Arthur Rank
Screenplay	Michael Powell, Emeric Pressburger
Photography	Jack Cardiff
Editor	Reginald Mills
Art Director	Alfred Jünge
Music	Allan Gray
Special Effects	Douglas Woolsey, Henry Harris

Cast

Peter Carter	David Niven
June	Kim Hunter

---

36 Haslam D. Medical classics: M*A*S*H. *BMJ*. 2007; **334**: 47.

| Dr Frank Reeves | Roger Livesey |
| Conductor 71 | Marius Goring |

REGENERATION (1997)

Credits

Director	Giles Mackinnon
Producers	Allan Scott, Peter R Simpson
Production Companies	Radford Films, BBC Films, Telefilm Canada, Glasgow Film Fund
Screenplay	Allan Scott
Original novel	Pat Barker
Photography	Glen Macpherson
Editor	Pia Di Ciaula
Art Director	John Frankish
Music	Mychael Danna

Cast

Dr William Rivers	Jonathan Pryce
Siegfried Sassoon	James Wilby
Billy Prior	Jonny Lee Miller
Wifred Owen	Stuart Bunce
Sarah	Tanya Allen
Dr Bryce	David Hayman
Robert Graves	Dougray Scott
Dr Yealland	John Neville
Dr Brock	Paul Young

DIVE BOMBER (1941)

Credits

Director	Michael Curtiz
Producer	Hal B Wallis
Production Company	Warner Bros
Screenplay	Frank Wead, Robert Buckner
Photography	Bert Glennon, Winton Hoch
Editor	George Amy
Art Director	Robert Haas
Music	Max Steiner
Special Effects	Byron Haskin, Rex Wimpy

Cast

| Lt Doug Lee, MD | Errol Flynn |
| Lt Cmdr Lance Rogers, MD | Ralph Bellamy |

| Lt Cmdr Joe Blake | Fred MacMurray |
| Mrs Linda Fisher | Alexis Fisher |

M*A*S*H (1970)

Credits

Director	Robert Altman
Producer	Ingo Preminger
Production Company	Twentieth Century Fox
Screenplay	Ring Lardner Jr
Original novel	Richard Hooker
Photography	Harry Stine
Editor	Danford B Greene
Art Directors	Jack Martin Smith, Arthur Lonergan
Music	Johnny Mandel

Cast

'Hawkeye' Pierce	Donald Sutherland
'Trapper John' McIntyre	Elliot Gould
Duke Forrest	Tom Skerritt
Colonel Henry Blake	Roger Bowen
Radar O'Reilly	Gary Burghoff
Major Frank Burns	Robert Duvall
Major Margaret Houlihan	Sally Kellerman
Father Mulcahy	Rene Auberjonois

CHAPTER 8

Wild Strawberries

John Salinsky

On a personal note

When I was a medical student in the early 1960s, I was fortunate to have friends in the Arts faculties who were enthusiastic about the latest films from Europe, and who dragged me along to see them. We saw films that were totally different from anything we had experienced before, and not just because they had subtitles. Over a curry afterwards we discussed our favourite directors – Renoir, Truffaut, Buñuel, Antonioni, Fellini and, of course, Ingmar Bergman. Along with its predecessor *The Seventh Seal*, Bergman's *Wild Strawberries* made a lasting impression on me. I never tire of seeing it, and there are scenes that still move me deeply.

Thirty years later, I started thinking about good films to show to trainee GPs. I wanted films that were classics – the best that cinema had to offer. I wanted them to have something serious to say about human relationships. Preferably they would be in black and white and in a foreign language with subtitles. They did not have to be about doctors, but the presence of a doctor in the story lent some respectability to my plan to show full-length films in an afternoon officially dedicated to medical education.

So *Wild Strawberries* was the perfect choice for my first film. The central character is a retired doctor who reflects on his life during the course of a journey to collect an honorary degree. The film is beautifully shot in black and white with dialogue in Swedish, and the cast are all brilliant. It is a masterpiece, I loved it and I wanted to share it.

About the director

Ingmar Bergman was born in 1918 in Uppsala and was brought up in Stockholm, where his father was a very strict Lutheran pastor. Bergman devoted his professional life to the theatre and the cinema, and became internationally famous in the 1960s for his serious, intense, lyrical films. Some people found their subject matter and symbolism hard going, but they were always beautifully acted and photographed. Bergman was able to resist the lure of Hollywood, and continued to work in Sweden with a small family of talented actors and technicians. His films are often close studies of relationships – between men and women, parents and children, brothers and sisters. By his own admission, they are mostly explorations of himself, and *Wild Strawberries* is no exception. He has been a great influence on younger directors, notably Woody Allen, who greatly admires Bergman and frequently pays him the compliment of imitation. Great films from his later career include *Persona, Cries and Whispers, Fanny and Alexander* and *Scenes from a Marriage*. His last film, *Sarabande*, was made in 2003 when he was 85 years of age. He died peacefully in his sleep on 30 July 2007, and the world of cinema mourned the passing of one of its greatest artists.

Unspooling the story

I shall now give you an outline of the story of *Wild Strawberries*, in order to refresh the memories of readers who know the film, and to give those who are not familiar with it an idea of what we are talking about.

The principal character is a 78-year-old emeritus professor of bacteriology, played by Victor Sjöström, who was one of the great directors of silent cinema in Sweden. The professor's name is Isak Borg, which roughly translated means 'Ice Fortress', giving us a clue to the frozen state of his emotions. However, as he introduces himself in voice-over and shows us round his sitting room, he seems amiable enough. He lives with his austere but devoted elderly housekeeper (Miss Agda), and is about to undertake a journey to the university city of Lund. There he will be honoured with the award of *Jubeldoktor* or 'Jubilee Doctor' in recognition of his 50 years of academic distinction. On the night before the journey he has a very disturbing dream about death, which is rendered in a chilling expressionist style. The next morning, to Miss Agda's dismay, he decides to travel the 600 kilometres from Stockholm by car instead of by air. He is accompanied by his daughter-in-law Marianne (played by the lovely and accomplished Ingrid Thulin). This journey takes up most of the film, so *Wild Strawberries* can claim to be one of the first road movies. Isak and Marianne talk about her failing marriage, and she tells him that he has a cold personality and apparently no human feelings – just like his son, her husband. He is intrigued rather than offended, perhaps because he is already beginning to reflect on what has been missing from his life. We realise now that he has also embarked on the Inner Journey, indispensable in a good road movie. On the way they stop at several places of significance in Isak's life. Near his parents' summer house he identifies his 'Wild Strawberry Patch' (of which more later). This triggers a daydream or reverie in which the old man slips back 60 years and eavesdrops on his adolescent sweetheart and cousin, Sara, as she picks wild strawberries and half reluctantly allows herself to be kissed by cousin Sigfrid, Isak's more confident elder brother. There follows a delightful scene in which we are able to watch Isak's large family (nine brothers and sisters) at breakfast as they celebrate deaf Uncle Aron's name day. Isak is woken from this dream by the arrival of a young student called Sara who reminds him of his cousin Sara. This is not surprising, as they are both very attractively played by Bibi Andersson, another member of Bergman's regular company, who also played a large part in the director's personal life. Sara is on her way to Italy with two young men, and Isak offers them a lift. Later on, they pick up a quarrelling couple (it is a very large car), who are subsequently ejected on to the road by Marianne because she cannot tolerate their spiteful behaviour. They stop for petrol in a village where the young Isak had worked as a GP for 15 years. The man who fills the car up greets his old family doctor very warmly and refuses to take any money. Isak wonders whether he should have remained a GP. They have an enjoyable *al fresco* lunch with the students. He and Marianne visit Isak's 96-year-old mother, another emotionally frozen person. As the journey continues, the students provide some welcome light relief and help to keep up the connection with youth. Sara flirts endearingly with the old man, who returns her affectionate joking. He nods off in the car while Marianne is driving, and has a horrible dream about taking a viva exam (which will bring a frisson of nightmarish recollection to anyone who has been a medical student). The examiner takes him out to the woods and shows him a vision of his late wife laughing mockingly as she has sex with her grinning wolfish lover. He wakes with a start and has a serious discussion with his daughter-in-law, who tells him that she is pregnant and determined to keep the baby, against her husband's wishes. By now the old man has learned how to listen and has begun to get in touch with his warmer feelings. They arrive in Lund, the degree ceremony takes place and the admiring students serenade him with a farewell song. Sara tells him that he is her only true love as she waves goodbye. He talks to his son, his daughter-in-law and Miss Agda. He then falls asleep, and dreams of greeting his parents as they sit by the lake at the old summer house, his father fishing. He smiles in his sleep, and seems to feel that when the time comes, he will die a little happier. This is the end of the movie.

I have been enthralled as much as ever. I want to see it again.

Victor Sjöström: a grand old man

Perhaps the most memorable and wonderful thing about *Wild Strawberries* is the performance of Victor Sjöström as Isak Borg. Sjöström had advised Bergman on directing the actors in his first film, and Bergman regarded him as something of a father figure. When he played Isak he was himself aged 78 years and rather frail, but it is a masterly and obviously deeply felt performance. There are many close-ups in which we can watch the emotions passing across his face like rapidly changing weather. And what a face! It is wrinkled, craggy, monumental, endearing and engaging. Apparently the 78-year-old veteran and the 22-year-old Bibi Andersson developed a tender, flirtatious relationship during the shooting which is also present in their interaction on the screen. Isak's relationships with the other women in his life are also fascinating, and we shall return to that subject a little later.

That car

The professor's car is an impressive presence, and it is an important character in the film. It is, I am reliably informed, a 1937 Packard Twelve Limousine which could hold up to seven people, if you opened up the 'jump seats' in the middle. As Isak tells Sara, 'It is an antique, like its owner.' You may notice that although the Packard is an American car with left-hand drive, it is driven on the left-hand side of the road. This is because in 1957 Sweden had yet to change over to driving on the right like the rest of continental Europe. Most of the car scenes were shot in the studio with back-projected scenery; but the story is so engrossing that I cease to notice this after the first few seconds.

Why is the film called *Wild Strawberries*?

I thought you were never going to ask. In fact the Swedish title *Smultronstället* means 'The Wild Strawberry Patch', which would sound a bit clumsy in English. I have already made several references to the wild strawberry patch in the woods which takes Isak back 60 years into a daydream vision of his sweetheart Sara, pretty and graceful in her summer dress, picking wild strawberries for Uncle Aron. In Swedish culture, wild strawberry patches in the woods have a special significance. Every child likes to have his or her own personal patch, which then comes to symbolise a special childhood memory, usually of summer, that its grown-up owner would like to revisit or recreate. So now it all makes sense, doesn't it?

Style of filming

Although it is a black-and-white film, the print available on DVD has a refreshing clarity with all of the detail visible. The scenes in the country convey the bright daylight of a Swedish summer. The woodland scenes from childhood are very lyrical, with light filtering through the leaves. Bergman uses shots of clouds, tree branches and birds to signal dramatic changes of mood in his characteristic way. The family breakfast scene is also brightly and cheerfully lit. Other scenes are more sombre (the examination dream, the sex-in-the-forest flashback, and Marianne's painful conversation with her husband in a smaller car, which takes place in the rain). Bergman uses many close-ups and 'two-shots' with which he is able to concentrate our attention on the characters' feelings as they speak. I often wonder to what extent the visual style of a film is determined by the vision of the director or the artistry of the cinematographer (in this case Gunnar Fischer, Bergman's regular collaborator in his early work). Probably it is the result of close partnership and sympathy between the two.

However, the remarkable structure of *Wild Strawberries* must be attributed to Bergman alone. It is very complicated, although this may not be apparent when you are caught up in the narrative. Isak introduces his story with a voice-over, but this device is used only sparingly in the rest of the film. His setting of the scene is rapidly followed or interrupted by the extended nightmare sequence, shot in high contrast and owing a great deal to German expressionism. He sees himself wandering in a strange deserted street, encountering a man without a face, and watching, paralysed with fear as a horse-drawn funeral carriage keels over, releasing the coffin which breaks open to reveal . . . himself. We are in no doubt that the prospect of death is dominating Isak's thoughts. The main narrative thread of the film is the car journey to Lund, but this is frequently interrupted by further dreams, reflections, reveries or whatever we like to call them. There are several 'flashbacks' to his young days. These are not, strictly speaking, memories, because his role is that of a time-travelling observer of scenes at which he was not present but that he somehow knows all about. We see Isak as an old man, invisible to the other characters, observing the events at Uncle Aron's name-day breakfast. This tableau has been serially recreated by Woody Allen, notably in *Annie Hall* and *Crimes and Misdemeanors*. In those films the families are of course Jewish American rather than Swedish, but the device of the grown-up observer visiting his childhood is the same. Later on, Isak sleeps in the car and goes into a long dream sequence, which starts with another encounter with young cousin Sara and leads to the unpleasant viva examination and the vision of his wife's infidelity. There is a final brief visit to that summer holiday of his adolescence before the film ends. Yes, the structure is complicated, but for me the interplay between present and past and between dream and reality only adds to the mystery and richness of the experience.

Now about those women . . .

It is time to discuss Professor Borg's relationships with the various female characters in his life. Bergman's films are famously full of beautiful actresses. The director himself was married five times, and also had love affairs with distinguished members of his company, including Bibi Andersson. He even made a film called *Now About These Women* (1962). In *Wild Strawberries*, the first woman we meet is Miss Agda, the professor's housekeeper. These two old folk play at being married while being careful to observe the proprieties. They bicker constantly and go into sulks, but are clearly very fond of each other. Then, rather to our surprise, the professor is joined by his daughter-in-law Marianne (played by Ingrid Thulin). We wonder what she is doing in the house. Marianne tells the old man very directly that she thinks that, behind his veneer of affability, he is cold and heartless. And yet, as their journey continues, the presence of the three young students seems to infuse both of them with some warmth, and they begin to like each other. Ingrid Thulin was 28 years old at the time of filming, and her calm beauty is awe-inspiring.

Then comes Bibi Andersson in her dual role as the two Saras. As Isak's cousin and secret fiancée in 1890 she has an irresistible pouting charm as she gathers strawberries and tries not to succumb to the advances of her randy cousin Sigfrid. When she confides in her older cousin Charlotta about the personalities of the two boys, we get an idea of why it was that Isak failed to hang on to her. Isak is serious and wants to read poetry or play duets together; but 'Sigrid is so fresh and exciting – and I want to go home!' Cousin Sara's difficulty in choosing between the two brothers is echoed by the modern Sara's indecision about the rival merits of her two student boyfriends. Sara, in her two manifestations, is the heart and soul of the picture and the source of the flame that warms the old man back to life.

Isak's 96-year-old mother is a formidable old lady; she has had nine children (all of whom are now dead except for Isak), and she has many grandchildren. However, she gets very few visits and, given her frigid manner, it is not hard to see why. We wonder what sort of motherly love Isak could possibly have received from her. And yet, when he and Marianne are anxious to cut short the visit, she wants them to stay. Under her thick layer of frost she, too, is lonely.

Finally, there is Isak's deceased wife, who appears in the flashback scene where he witnesses her infidelity in the forest. Her mocking laughter as she succumbs to her lover's assaults seems to be aimed at her husband. She knows that he will forgive her, she says, but we get the impression that this is only because he doesn't really care. Isak's wife seems to be there to show us that his marriage was a miserable failure. But how much is this his fault? We learn from Alman, the 'examiner', that she has accused him of indifference, selfishness, and lack of consideration. At the end of the sequence when Mrs Borg disappears, he congratulates Isak ironically on having surgically excised her: 'everything has been dissected, Professor Borg. A surgical masterpiece. There is no pain, no bleeding, no quivering.' Isak asks what the penalty is, to which he receives the reply 'The usual one . . . loneliness.' Alman appears earlier as the male half of the quarrelling couple who have to be ejected from the car. So he seems to know all about failed marriages.

Discussion of the Borgs' marriage leads us on to a consideration of their son Evald, Marianne's husband. We learn that he is also a professor of medicine and, although only 38 years of age, he is already cold and remote, just like his father. He expects no warmth from the old man, and receives none. The only support that he has received is a loan which he is determined to pay back. Gratitude is not something he can afford.

The final scene between Isak, Evald and Marianne seems to offer a slender hope that Evald will be reunited with Marianne and that he will accept the role of father to their child. However, I wouldn't put a lot of money on it.

Problems and difficulties

Are there any scenes in the film that don't work? There are certainly some that jar and cause discomfort. For me these include the two 'scenes from a marriage' (the title of Bergman's later film which was made initially as a series for television). I find the sneering, sarcastic exchanges of the Almans in the car acutely painful and even embarrassing. They seem to have been ripped too violently from Bergman's personal experiences without enough artistic transformation. The almost-rape adultery in the forest with the wife's hideous laughter also makes me squirm because of its rawness, but perhaps that is Bergman's intention. Then there is the whole question of the mock viva. The build-up in which a dignified old professor is subjected to a public oral examination in front of the three students who admire him so much is perfect in its horrible humiliation. And I love the microscope that only reflects the eye of the beholder. But then the candidate is asked to read some incomprehensible printed letters on the blackboard. It is not English, and we soon realise that it is not Swedish either. There are echoes of the writing on the wall that mystified Belshazzar and informed him he had been 'weighed in the balance and found wanting.' Alman tells Isak that on the blackboard is written 'the first duty of a doctor.' Isak is expected to remember this as if it was the Hippocratic Oath, but fails to do so. We all get a shock when Alman tells him that 'the first duty of a doctor is to ask forgiveness.' What is that all about? Furthermore, the old man is told that he is 'guilty of guilt' and has been judged 'incompetent.' We seem to have strayed into Kafka territory. Presumably he is guilty of lack of emotional competence, but I don't find this scene very convincing. However, these flaws, if such they be, are a small price to pay for all the delights of the rest of the film.

Favourite scenes

There are so many of these from which to choose. I would have to include all of the scenes featuring Miss Agda, a stout, dignified little person who is admirably played by Jullan Kindahl. I love it when she impatiently takes over from her boss's clumsy attempt to pack his own suitcase, and he stands back and says smarmily 'There is no one who can pack like you.' She responds drily 'Is that so?', and he mutters 'Old sourpuss!'

Then, when we stop by the wild strawberry patch and cousin Sara appears with her basket, like a vision of spring, I dissolve completely. I am captivated by her indignation when she scolds her amorous cousin Sigfrid: 'Besides, the twins who know *everything* say that you've been doing *bad things* with the Berglund girl. And she's not a *really nice* girl, the twins say. And I believe them.' I look forward to seeing the twins in person, sitting round the breakfast table and chanting in unison 'Sigfrid and Sara! Sigfrid and Sara!', until the distraught Sara rushes out in confusion to be comforted by Charlotta as Isak looks on and wishes that he had taken the plunge when he had the chance.

I am always moved (for some reason) by the affection and respect that the three students have for the old man. Their love and their liveliness seem to help him to recover his humanity. Ingrid Thulin's performance as Marianne wins more admiration from me every time I see it. And Victor Sjöström's face in close-up is always wonderful to behold. Finally, I like that final long shot of the old man's parents waving to him from beside the lake. I have often noticed that as old people get closer to death their need to get in touch with their inner parents becomes urgent.

Inner meanings?

I do not in the least want to be accused of reductionism, but what is *Wild Strawberries* really all about? Bergman has said that in many of his films he is confronting one of his own fears. Here the theme of regret about emotional coldness, and the wish to overcome it, is very evident. This is brought out in the treatment of Isak's early loss of Sara and his subsequent failed marriage. And what about his relationship with his gloombag son Evald, who cannot even crack a smile when his wife tells him she is pregnant? We know from his autobiographical writings that the young Bergman had to endure humiliation and frequent beatings from his own father, who was tyrannical and emotionally distant. He also said that in *Wild Strawberries* he wanted to 'justify myself to mythically oversized parents.' Does Isak Borg represent Bergman's father? I have already suggested that Victor Sjöström, the veteran director, was a kind of father figure. However, it is more complicated than that, because it seems that in taking on the role Sjöström was also dealing with his own inner demons. Philip and Kersti French, in their excellent BFI monograph on the film (French and French, 1995), quote Ingmar Bergman writing as follows:

> Victor Sjöström took my text, made it his own, invested it with his own experiences: his pain, his misanthropy, his brutality, sorrow, fear, loneliness, coldness, warmth, hardness and ennui. Borrowing my father's form he occupied my soul and made it all his own . . .
>
> (Bergman, 1994)

Is there a message for doctors?

The main message is the one about staying in touch with your feelings. Doctors cannot hear that too often, and it comes over better in a work of art than in a lecture or a textbook. Don't use your profession as a way of escaping from life, the film tells us. In life as in medicine, pain is nature's way of telling us that there is something wrong, and it is no good applying a layer of ice to the affected part without exploring what is going on underneath. However, even if you are a hardened case, like Professor Borg, redemption is possible – but don't leave it too late! Remember how much your patients love you (remember the scene at the petrol pump), which shows that underneath that protective carapace there beats a human heart. And for goodness sake let us get rid of those terrible viva exams. I think that is about it for the official messages. Unofficially I would like all doctors and students to be given the opportunity to see *Wild Strawberries* so that at least some of them will experience the lasting pleasure it has given me and thousands of others. Then they will know that it exists and can be remembered and revisited (like the *smultronstället*) whenever they feel the need.

References

Bergman I. *Images* (translated by Marianne Ruuth). London: Bloomsbury; 1994.
French P, French K. *Wild Strawberries*. BFI Film Classics. London: British Film Institute; 1995.

Filmography

SMULTRONSTÄLLET (WILD STRAWBERRIES) 1957

Credits

Production Company	Svensk Filmindustri
Director	Ingmar Bergman
Screenplay	Ingmar Bergman
Photography	Gunnar Fischer

Cast

Professor Isak Borg	Victor Sjöström
Miss Agda	Jullan Kindahl
Marianne Borg	Ingrid Thulin
Sara, a student/Sara, Isak's cousin	Bibi Andersson
Stan Alman, an engineer	Gunnar Sjöberg
Berit Alman, his wife	Gunnel Broström
Dr Evald Borg, Isak's son	Gunnar Björnstrand
Isak's mother	Nalma Wifstrand
Harold Akerman, petrol station owner	Max von Sydow

CHAPTER 9

Real lives. I: A series of awakenings

A long time ago in a faraway land – Russia in the 1920s – a folklorist with the Beckettian name of Propp argued that the hundreds of fairy stories of his country were all constructed from a fixed set of narrative functions and were played out by a fixed set of main characters – the number of each being 31 and 7, respectively (Propp, 1928). Although some may baulk at what seems like reductive quantification in the face of creative diversity, the theory paves the way for important ideas – for instance, that things which appear dissimilar to the casual observer may have common roots (e.g. a modern hearing aid and the timing mechanism in a VW Golf, both of which rely on digital technology). Or, to follow the causal chain the other way, we can see how things might start from the same source and end up in very different places. Frenchman Raymond Queneau wrote a book called *Exercises de Style* (Queneau, 1947), which comprised 99 retellings of the same simple tale of a bus journey during which a couple of everyday incidents occur – one account is called 'Free verse', another is called 'Olfactory', a third 'Negativities', and so on. (The book was itself inspired by Bach's *Art of the Fugue*, perhaps the most famous musical exercise in themes and variations.) This chapter is in a similar vein, although mercifully it does not have 99 variations of anything.

Our starting point is a natural phenomenon that baffled the medical profession for most of the twentieth century,[37] namely the sleeping-sickness

---

[37] The only part of the twentieth century during which the phenomenon did not baffle the profession was in the 16 years before it occurred; for no proper understanding of it has ever been reached.

epidemic of 1916–27. This was not the infectious disease of the same name spread by the tsetse fly; but rather *encephalitis lethargica*, a viral inflammation of the brain that caused paralysis, behavioural disturbances and lethargy to the point of catatonia, among other symptoms. The scale of the epidemic was of the order of 5 million people worldwide, of whom around a third died during its decade-long reign of terror. The disease then disappeared as inexplicably as it had arrived; and, some individual or small-scale incidences notwithstanding, it has not come back since.

Enter Oliver Sacks, now world famous as an author and neurologist, but simply a young doctor in 1966 when he joined the staff at Beth Abraham, a chronic mental hospital in a suburb of New York. There he encountered an accumulation of survivors of the epidemic, an 80-strong cohort who had been largely forgotten (in research and treatment terms). The situation – of a rich historical natural phenomenon lying dormant right in front of him – was irresistible for a man of Sacks' enquiring nature, and he became deeply involved with the patients and their disease. He wrote up his experiences in a book called *Awakenings* (Sacks, 1973).

The book

The book's title derives from a particular period – the summer months of 1969 – when, under the influence of a drug treatment initiated by Sacks, the patients seemed to awaken from their years of sleeping sickness, and recovered something approaching a normal 'healthy' state. That is to say, people who had been lost for decades in their private worlds of mental sickness, who had been more or less incommunicado, started to interact in an articulate, self-aware way, reflecting on what had happened to them and discussing it with healthcare staff and with each other. However, the drug's benefits proved to be short-lived, and were soon accompanied by problematic side-effects; and so a resumption of the previous status quo gradually occurred.

Sacks' account of the events is, self-consciously, something more than a medical report and something less than a 'storified' version of events. Twenty case histories (discrete mini-stories) form the core of the book; but they come topped and tailed by contextualising sections that provide scientific, historical and social information, as well as Sacks' own broader 'metaphysical' (his term) musings prompted by the extraordinary phenomena that he witnessed. These latter have chapter headings such as 'Tribulation' and 'Accommodation.' Sacks also describes the resistance with which his work was met by the medical community, a classic case study for sociologists interested in epistemological paradigm shifts.

The book itself has appeared in several editions since its original publication, in each of which Sacks has added or subtracted significant material; and so it could be said to be several different entities in itself.

The TV documentary

The appearance of the book was soon followed by a 45-minute-long documentary made for UK television (Yorkshire TV, 1973), also called *Awakenings*. Of course, documentaries come in a range of shapes and sizes – think of the difference between *Fahrenheit 9/11* (Michael Moore, 2003) and *Être et Avoir* (Nicolas Philibert, 2003) – and this one falls somewhere in the middle of the spectrum. That is to say, there is an unseen, voice-over narrator who links around 40 scenes. The latter include shots of newspaper cuttings of the time (the 1920s); interviews with Sacks (during which he does some disconcertingly good imitations of his patients' physical tics), the patients and their relatives; and clips from Sacks' own movies (i.e. 'home' movies), shot over several years in the hospital.

The programme reaches the halfway stage (the point when it breaks for commercials) at what Sacks calls the 'time of elation', when the drug seemed to be working and there were hopes that a miracle cure had been effected. The second half, which has fewer (and therefore longer) scenes than the first, charts the decline of the patients. Notwithstanding this, the programme ends on a balanced note (in terms of emotional affect), wherein the state of sickness is conferred with if not a certain nobility then at least a dignified honesty. It shows how the events did not culminate in the awakenings – perfect happy-ever-after outcome though this would have been – but rather in a greater ability of many of the patients (and staff) to come to terms with the disease. (Several of them were maintained on low-dose drug treatment, and experienced life with partial lucidity. The programme includes interviews with some of them in this halfway-house state.)

The play

Sacks' title was inspired by that of an Ibsen play, and in 1982 the story was reclaimed by the theatre via a work by Harold Pinter (Pinter, 1982). Pinter has produced a large body of writing, not all of it for the stage; but much of his theatrical output is characterised by the portrayal of fractured relationships between one person and another, or between one person and the world around them. The effect is to present normally concealed elements of the mind for inspection, and through this (and Pinter's particularly fine ear for phraseology) to convey a sense of displacement, an experience of seeing things from a different and bracing perspective. Even from such a simplified sketch of his artistic style, it should be clear how the world that Sacks depicts in *Awakenings* might have seemed to Pinter like off-the-peg material for one of his plays. (Pinter's poetic title, *A Kind of Alaska*, is almost sufficient as QED.)

The play is short (35 pages of text and not as many minutes in performance) and takes place in one scene in a room with two characters and then a third. These are a female patient, a male doctor, and then the patient's sister (who is also the doctor's wife). The action, such as it is, consists of the patient having an 'awakening' experience followed by what seem to be the first stages of a slide back towards sickness. However, it is the dialogue that counts; and Pinter uses it to juxtapose past and present in such a way that the poignancy of time passing, and the fact that all lives are lived irrevocably, is keenly felt by the audience. There is much that is memorably expressed. For example, the patient says of her lost years 'I've been dancing in very narrow spaces'; and her doctor (who has become emotionally entangled with her to the detriment of his marriage) is the one who describes her once-removed, pre-awakened mental state as like living in 'a kind of Alaska.'

The film

At 121 minutes, the film is substantially longer than either the TV documentary or the play. This gives it room to expand, like the book. It begins with an extended prelude that fades to black at the end of the credits, wherein a young boy called Leonard Lowe is seen gradually succumbing to a disease that effectively 'freezes' him (i.e. drastically reduces his motor functions). The time and setting are established approximately by visual information (e.g. period clothes and cars, the Manhattan Bridge) as winter in New York in the 1920s. The film then cuts to a sunny, more modern urban setting (which we discover to be 1960s New York), as Dr Malcolm Sayer comes for an interview for a junior medical post at a psychiatric hospital. Because Sayer is played by Robin Williams (joint top-billed in the credits and a well-known actor) we take this to be a central character; and the effect is of a second beginning to the film, which we now assume to be about this medic. Similarly, because he too is joint top-billed and a well-known actor, we notice Robert De Niro in the background of various shots in the hospital, as he intermittently appears as one of a group of patients with whom we are becoming acquainted. However, it is some time and several significant plot points later before we realise that De Niro is the now adult Leonard, the opening vignette having been half forgotten during the development of the second (doctor) storyline. In due course, Sayer uses Lowe as the guinea pig in an experimental drug treatment. It proves successful, so it is extended to other patients in the group, who all benefit. However, Lowe regresses in increasingly antisocial stages until, at the end of the film, he has reverted to his former, semi-somnolent state. The other patients look on, knowing that they are likely to follow a similar path.

One classic Hollywood narrative is to have parallel storylines in which the hero overcomes an external enemy while negotiating obstacles to a heterosexual love affair. This film does not dispense with that formula, but tempers it in various significant ways:

➤ There are no serious (i.e. demonised or persistent) antagonists (in contrast, say, to *One Flew Over The Cuckoo's Nest* (Forman, 1973)). The only significant opposition that Sayer faces is the disease, notwithstanding his faintly patronising, slightly obstructive medical colleagues.

➤ The supposed miracle cure in the tradition of 'throw away the crutches and play the violin at Carnegie Hall' (to mix metaphors) proves to be a mirage. This itself is a challenge to the common American belief that simple power can cure all problems (medical or otherwise), as embodied by pharmaceutical solutions to ill health.

➤ The film ends on a resolutely downbeat, even regressive note in relation to the patients.

So there is no fundamental alteration of the patients' story as compared with the book, the documentary or the play (except that the play deals with one patient only); and indeed Sacks was involved in the film's production as medical adviser, and so is arguably some kind of guarantor. Perhaps this is because facts as strange as those relating to the 'Awakenings phenomenon' are like manna for storytellers in general and Hollywood in particular, because they sanction the use of the expression 'based on a true story.' This phrase instantly allays the doubts about realism that are intrinsic to all artworks, while enabling exciting (in the sense of 'less dull than perceived ordinary life') stories to be told.[38]

---

38 Sacks has said that he would have written his book even if there had been no awakenings, because of the fascination of a disease which assumed many forms and of

Nonetheless, of course, the film differs from other versions, and we shall consider three of the important ways in which it does so.

The first is the greatly enlarged role of the doctor, as touched on earlier, for the film is as much about Sayer's awakening as it is about Lowe's. He moves from a starting point of immersion – even submersion – in the world of recondite natural science, and extreme social gaucheness ('geekiness', one could say), to being able to ask a female colleague out on something approaching a date.[39] This progress is explicitly linked to his exposure to the patients (especially Lowe) and their lust for a life that includes human interaction; as well as to his socio-political engagement in the fight for the patients' well-being in the face of an uninterested medical staff (an anti-establishment issue that we have noted in Sacks' book), although this is probably fuelled as much by his belief in scientific truth as by any craving for social (i.e. altruistic) justice.

The scene in which Lowe awakens is emblematic. This event might have been shown as an immense personal transformation – a kind of Jekyll-and-Hyde moment in reverse. Instead, it is presented as a low-volume exercise in tension and release, and a shared triumph. The trial drug has been showing little effect, and Sayer keeps edging up the dosage in consultation with the hospital pharmacist, his reputation (not to mention his fragile self-image) at stake; until one night he takes the radical step of unilaterally quadrupling the quantity administered. He settles down to observe Lowe; but as the night wears on, and with the patient showing no sign of a reaction, he falls asleep on his watch, propped up in Lowe's bedside wheelchair. He wakes up some time later and the camera pulls back to show Lowe's bed alongside him, now empty. Sayer, startled, walks off in search of the hitherto immobile patient and finds him sitting in the adjacent day-room, bent over a table. Lowe's position makes it hard to tell whether he is 'frozen' or not. As Sayer approaches him, Lowe looks up slowly, his expression blank as if he is still as absent as ever. Then the slightest of smiles plays upon his lips, and he mumbles a word: 'Quiet.' Sayer cautiously replies 'It's late – everyone's asleep.' Lowe,

---

patients who all coped differently with it. One cannot see Hollywood doing the same, though; or maybe it would have set the story in 1916–27, instead of 1967; because it is the patients' proximity to normality that makes the events so anguishing. If there was no hope of recovery, an audience might not be very moved – or perhaps it would be moved by the healthy relatives, or the patient at the point when he felt that he was losing his hold on the real world. Indeed, this 'proximity to normality' is the common hook in all versions.

39 An act that lightens the film's otherwise downbeat ending noted earlier.

his smile slowly broadening, says, 'I'm not asleep!'; to which Sayer answers 'No – you're awake . . .'; as he too breaks into a wide smile. De Niro's skilfully calibrated expressivity ensures that Sayer (like the cinema audience) is kept in suspense as to his condition for as long as possible. And the evident role overlap between the two men – consider Williams in Lowe's wheelchair asleep while Lowe is taking steps towards rejoining the human race – is understated but powerful. The scene ends with the two men sharing the joy of realisation of what has just happened, this being an equally momentous event for both of them.

A second distinguishing feature of the film is perhaps self-evident, yet no less important for that, namely that it is a mainstream movie and therefore brings to bear the well-established techniques of that medium. Hollywood goes to tremendous lengths to mount its productions in a way that the broad movie-going public has come to accept as normal. It invests time and money on costumes and lighting, on camera angles and editing, on accompanying music and so on – that is to say, on all the paraphernalia of cinematography. This tends to 'make presentable' all that it alights on, and a story that is told utilising these means is experienced very differently to the same story told in the theatre or in a TV documentary, let alone on the printed page, to the extent that it is almost not the same story. For instance, the carefully timed introduction of music in the 'awakening' scene that has just been described, and the measured use of shot-countershot[40] at its climax, push the audience's interpretation of the action in certain directions.

If the second criterion for comparison risks being underestimated because it is so manifest, there is a third that appears equally obvious in theory but proves far harder to elucidate in practice, namely the attribution of authorship, and its effect on the finished product. The film version of *Awakenings* (1990) had apparently been languishing in development limbo until it was seized upon by Penny Marshall, who produced and directed the film. This gives her a prima facie claim to being the creative vision behind the project. However, the variables that shape what Hollywood likes to call 'a major motion picture' are numerous and complicated, and notoriously difficult to disentangle. For instance, co-producer Walter Parkes stated that 'Penny has really commercial instincts, populist instincts. She'd open it [i.e. the movie of the book *Awakenings*] up rather than make it too cerebral or arty' (*Premiere*,

---

40 A standard way of filming a two-way conversation, in which each speaker dominates the frame in turn.

p. 90) – the possible inference being that were it otherwise, funding might not have been forthcoming. (Apparently, one studio suggestion was to turn Sayer or Lowe into a woman so that the two characters could have a love affair!) Artistically, too, Marshall did not exert total control, allowing director of photography Miroslav Ondricek to 'take care of me [while] I try to deal with the actors' (*Premiere*, p. 90). Ondricek has explained how he attempted to tell the story photographically – for instance, by ensuring that the lighting gradually became richer and warmer as the story moved towards the patients' halcyon awakened days. This plurality, which is endemic to the making of all films to a greater or lesser extent, might be seen as a bonus (Ondricek is a widely respected cameraman) or as a dire threat to the integrity of a work of art (because commercial pressures usually equate with corny values); and it supports the instinctive feeling that something written by the eminent Dr Oliver Sacks or Harold Pinter (a Nobel prize winner) or filmed as a documentary must somehow be 'superior' to a Hollywood movie. And yet the film of *Awakenings* conveys many points that are present in Sacks' original book very effectively, precisely because it contextualises those points slightly differently. It also subtracts and adds points. So perhaps artistic provenance can be seen as a red herring in relation to quality, and we should replace it with something more audience-centred – the notion of personal taste, perhaps. The 'best' version then becomes the one that pleases a given spectator or reader most, for whatever reasons.[41]

Another word of caution – it is important to realise that considering this set of artefacts (i.e. *Awakenings* in all of its forms) from a comparative perspective may lead to the downplaying of other elements that it contains. For instance, one commentator has seen Pinter's play as part of a bigger story of gender battles acted out in his work (Ham, 1993); and acting students could discuss the film in the context of De Niro's recurrent interest in outsiders, ranging from Travis Bickle in *Taxi Driver* (Scorsese, 1976) to Frankenstein's monster in *Mary Shelley's Frankenstein* (Branagh, 1994); and so on. There are many ways to cut a cake.

Closing thoughts

It can be argued that all narrative art is realistic at source (i.e. it is 'based on a true story'), whether it originates in the internal reality of an artist's

---

41 This debate about highbrow vs. lowbrow and objectivity vs. subjectivity is unlikely to be resolved until after Man has discovered the meaning of life.

imagination or in events taking place in more public domains. The artist then opts for more or less mimetic (i.e. imitative as opposed to transformative) ways of communicating this realism. Munch's *The Scream* does not much resemble the physical world, yet most people can recognise existential (and so 'realistic') truths in the painting. We tend to focus on storylines in the narrative arts such as literature, film and theatre, just as we focus on melody in music; so if someone asks us about a film that we have seen, the first thing we will tell them is the plot. The aim of this chapter has been to try to wean us off this reflex response, if only temporarily; and to illustrate how different people can do a very different 'show and tell', even though they are using the same basic materials. The *International Classification of Diseases* attempts to categorise and so 'fix' diseases, and provides an invaluable starting point for diagnosis and treatment. However, we should think of Propp, and *Awakenings*, and remember that real life – or, more accurately, real individuals' lives – can rarely be categorised; and that their meaning is determined as much by context as by content. The skill is to discern which elements of a story are being privileged, and what significance this has for our response to it.

References

Abramowitz R. *Premiere (US edition)*. 1991; **4**: 88–91.
Cerner B. *American Cinematographer*. 1991; **2**: 26–9.
Ham MC. Portrait of Deborah: a kind of Alaska. In: Burkmann K, Kundert-Gibbs J (eds) *Pinter at Sixty*. Bloomington, IN: Indiana University Press; 1993.
Pinter H. *A Kind of Alaska*. London: Methuen; 1982.
Propp V. *Morphology of the Folk Tale*. Austin, TX: University of Texas Press; 1928.
Queneau R. *Exercises de Style*. Paris: Editions Gallimard; 1947.
Sacks O. *Awakenings*. New York: Vintage; 1973.

Filmography

AWAKENINGS (1990)

Credits

Director	Penny Marshall
Producers	Walter Parkes, Lawrence Lasker
Production Company	Columbia
Screenplay	Steven Zaillian
Original book	Oliver Sacks
Photography	Miroslav Ondricek
Editors	Jerry Greenberg, Battle Davis
Art director	Bill Groom

| Music | Randy Newman |
| Technical adviser | Oliver Sacks |

Cast

Dr Malcolm Sayer	Robin Williams
Leonard Lowe	Robert De Niro
Eleanor Costello	Julie Kavner
Dr Kaufman	John Heard
Mrs Lowe	Ruth Nelson

CHAPTER 10

Real lives. II: Biopics

In the last chapter we saw a group of patients and their doctor commandeered for artistic service, the film (and play and TV documentary and book) about them shaped into a story around a circumscribed series of events. Now we shall turn our attention to a different, generic instance of film-makers pinning the 'true story' badge on their lapel – the biopic. Biopics are tales of men (and occasionally women) who are famous for one thing or another, be it performing popular songs (as in *Walk the Line* (Mangold, 2006), about country-and-western star Johnny Cash), or inventing the naturalist novel (*The Life of Emile Zola* (Dieterle, 1937)), or promoting insurgency (*Lawrence of Arabia* (Lean, 1962)). The first flowering of the genre took place in the late 1930s and 1940s. In those days the films were usually elevating, and some of the most famous examples involved doctors, whether of the PhD or medical variety. *Dr Ehrlich's Magic Bullet* (Dieterle, 1940), which deals with the medic who discovered a cure for syphilis, is a model of its kind.

The film begins as it means to continue, the title sequence being appropriated to convey an early pro-science message. Behind the credits are a series of close-ups in silhouette of the arms or tilting head of a laboratory scientist going about his business – poring over slides, pouring liquids from one receptacle to another, and so on. There is no set (i.e. no backdrop), and the equipment – which is repeatedly reconfigured so as to discourage any attempts at spatial mapping by the viewer – seems to be on a free-standing workbench, an artificial space created by the film. The deliberate non-specificity of both the location and the human presence in it make this a symbolic representation of science and some of its cherished tenets – for instance, patience (the figure appears entirely unhurried), and suppression of ego in the interests of objectivity and replicability (both implied by the impersonality and framing of the silhouettes). The swelling orchestra on the soundtrack suggests that a story of import and drama will follow, and this sense is reinforced by an intertitle which follows the last credit: 'This picture is dedicated to Dr Paul Ehrlich, whose dream it was to create out of chemicals "Magic Bullets" with which to fight the scourges of mankind . . . and this is the story of his devotion to that ideal.' These are big words being bandied about ('dream', 'create out of chemicals', 'scourges of mankind', 'devotion' and 'ideal'), so it would appear that this Ehrlich guy is quite something.

The first scene is loaded with more orientating information. Dr Ehrlich is examining a patient, a callow youth who is plainly worried. Ehrlich is calm and kindly, but concludes that the patient's problem is serious, although it is not named ('What you have is a contagious disease, an infection like any other'). The patient says that he has a girlfriend he loves, and asks whether they will be able to marry. Ehrlich replies that marriage is out of the question (from which the audience can infer that the disease is sexually transmitted[42]). When the patient asks whether there is a cure, Ehrlich reassures him that there is – sweat baths; but cannot look him in the eye as he says this. As the patient goes into a changing cubicle in a corner of the room, a colleague of Ehrlich's (called Wolfert) comes in and complains that Ehrlich has not been keeping up to date with his paperwork. He is soon followed by a clerk, who pesters Ehrlich to sign some forms. Then a middle-aged patient who has been waiting outside puts his head through the open door to ask whether he can see Ehrlich. Ehrlich ushers him in, and on hearing that the sweat bath treatment is interfering with his ability to do his job, agrees that he can stop it. Again, Wolfert upbraids him – first, for running the clinic an hour beyond its official midday end-time; and secondly, for sanctioning the discontinuation of treatment:

'Our superior has ordered sweat baths in such cases.'

'You know as well as I do that they're of no value whatsoever. This is my patient – I don't see in what way it affects you, Dr Wolfert?'

'That's beside the point. A hospital is an organisation, and an organisation must have rules, and rules have to be obeyed by everyone.'

---

42 The word 'syphilis' is not used in the film, in order to avoid upsetting the censors. The very fact that the disease was central to the story was exceptionally bold for the time.

The argument is interrupted by a noise from the changing cubicle. The camera swish-pans to the young patient, who is lying prostrate on the floor at the foot of the cubicle curtains with an open razor in his hand and his wrist slashed. He has overheard the truth about the non-efficacy of treatment and has committed suicide.

So we have been shown several facets of Ehrlich's individuality – his patient-centred approach which is not in keeping with what is plainly the traditionally hierarchical institution in which he works; his non-judgmental stance in relation to his patients' diseases; his forgetfulness when it comes to humdrum bureaucracy; his stubbornness in the face of attempts to curb his autonomy; and his unease at the current limits of the scientific knowledge relating to 'scourges of mankind.' These are some of the ingredients identified by those who have written about medical biopics, such as Babington (2005) and Elena (1993), and others follow later in the film. Babington, having made the important point that the medical biopic should more properly be termed the medical *researcher* biopic, has demonstrated the almost slavish adherence in the films of this period, such as *Dr Ehrlich's Magic Bullet*, *The Life of Louis Pasteur* (1936, Dieterle) and *Madame Curie* (1943, LeRoy), to a recipe that includes 'a progressive individual fighting for enlightenment against an outmoded establishment; a narrative formed around a "trial" scene vindicating the protagonist'; a root in the nineteenth century (i.e. some 50 years before the film's production), so that 'the audience witness the creation of their own ameliorated conditions' (p. 121); and so on.

Meanwhile, Elena was the first to draw attention to the curious undertow of religious allusion in the film that coexists, counter-intuitively, with the promotion of secular (i.e. scientific and humanist) values – in particular, how the trajectory of the main protagonist's story seems to mirror the Epiphany, Passion and Ascension of Christ.

'If it works, don't fix it' is a sound commercial (and even artistic) axiom; and a winning formula was particularly attractive to Hollywood during that period at the height of the studio system. There were plenty of other examples of mass production, including one of a medical hue – ten Dr Kildare films were made in the five years between 1937 and 1942 (not for nothing was Hollywood called the 'dream *factory*'). However, as we have seen elsewhere in this book, there is often a wild card in the pack. In this instance, non-conformism comes in the shape of *The Great Moment*, made in 1944 by writer–director Preston Sturges. This film tells the story of William Morton, the Massachusetts man who has some claim to being the inventor of modern anaesthesia in 1848.

A corrosively satirical take on the medical researcher film, Sturges uses the format to savage the American Way and all who sail in her, just as he did from different angles in other films, such as *Sullivan's Travels* (1941). In *The Great Moment*, he debunks the Great Man Myth. Morton is portrayed as an ordinary fellow of no more than middling intelligence and competence who is driven as much by commercial necessity as by altruism. For a start, he is a failed medical student, who goes into dentistry as a second-best career. He sets up practice only for his very first patient to jump out of the chair and run away because of the pain of treatment. This being the 1840s, 'no patients' was directly equated with 'no income.'[43] So it is his own poverty that Morton wants to alleviate more than the patient's suffering when he tries to find a way of anaesthetising clients. (After his subsequent success in the field, he is shown living in a mansion with servants, and his wife entertaining lavishly.)

Further to this, the film highlights the difficulty of attributing ownership of intellectual property rather than promoting the cult of the individual genius. Morton's discovery of inhaled ether (which he calls letheon, after the River Lethe, the river of oblivion in Greek mythology) is aided by crucial if some-what haphazard contributions of others at various stages – in other words, scientific advances do not come out of nowhere (or one person's head), as most biopics imply.

Then there is the title itself. The 'great moment' is not, as might be expected, that of the discovery of a usable anaesthetic – it is the embracing of selflessness, even personal loss, for the benefit of others that Morton accedes to near the end of the film when he reveals the secret of his system in order to save a young servant girl from agony during an operation. There is no happy ending – indeed, it is this act of selflessness (which occurs in the context of an ongoing battle over patents) that is suggested as the root cause of Morton's early death. The film may sound irredeemably bleak, but in fact plays as a comedy for much of its running time. The march of science here incorporates chasing the Morton family's pet dog around the parlour to experiment on; while Morton's wife berates him for not attending to his domestic commit-ments, and threatens to go back to her mother (unlike the quietly supportive, long-suffering spouses of the classic model). Also, it is shot through with Sturges' signature mordant wit and sharp-as-a-tack dialogue (for example,

---

43 Although some may argue that things are not so different now.

when deciding what to call his new wonder drug, so as to protect his possibility of a patent, Morton says to his wife, 'I've thought of a pretty good name – did you ever hear of the River Lethe in mythology?'; to which she replies, 'I never even heard of mythology . . .'). All in all, the film is a wonderfully rich contemporary counterpoint to the prevailing template.

Biopics are in fashion these days too, of course; and three recent candidates for inclusion in the medical field are worth mentioning here. Chronologically, the first is *Breast Men* (1997), and it is the most difficult to classify. The title suggests that the film cannot be a biopic, since it promises to focus on more than one person – which is a little misleading, as it turns out. A more substantial objection is that its main protagonist is given a fictional name ('Kevin Saunders', standing approximately for the real-life Frank Gerow), a fact that probably restricts it to Associate Membership of the canon. And yet it should be in this chapter, at least. The film traces the story of a trainee medic who moves from obscurity to fame as a result of his medical innovation, which he has developed by the classic biopic components of against-the-grain ingenuity and trial and error. The fact that his 'discovery' was the silicone breast implant – with all of its attendant health risks – says much about how the world has 'progressed' since 1940 (even the trenchant critique in *The Great Moment* did not extend to questioning the benefits of anaesthesia). Saunders' motives are more self-centred than Morton's, let alone Ehrlich's (in their cinematic incarnations), and seem to originate at least in part from his own sense of personal and professional inadequacy. The story, in its bid to follow the path of the hapless protagonist, rides sideways across several tracks without ever properly addressing them (for example, the issue of women's self-image and its relationship to cultural norms, the ethical issues surrounding the customer-is-king (or in this case, queen) model when applied to certain branches of medicine, the intertwinement of medical research and pharmaceutical companies in the USA, and so on). From a film genre point of view, there is an element of documentary (thanks to a curious framing device) and a touch of body horror. However, taking the potpourri as a whole, it is a cautionary tale rather than a celebration of science – exchange Faust for Christ as the role model, or *Paradise Lost* for the New Testament as the source book – and so not an *echt* biopic.

If *Breast Men* sits uneasily on the edges of the genre, *The Motorcycle Diaries* (Salles, 2004) is firmly back with the last chapter's *Awakenings* (Marshall, 1990) as a drama based on relatively tightly delineated events (in fact its 'best-fit' genre is 'road movie', as the title implies), so is something of a red herring here, notwithstanding the high profile that it had on release. Again, however, it deserves mention in a chapter that deals with films about real-life doctors who have made a mark on the world. In this case, the tale is based on a journey taken around South America by the young Che Guevara, then halfway through medical school, during which his political conscience is born. Clearly, the main protagonist fits the criterion for a biopic in general, if that is that the central figure should be someone who has had an important impact on a strand of history. In its thematic material, though, the film has more in common with the social conscience pictures of the 1930s, such as *I Am a Fugitive from a Chain Gang* (LeRoy, 1932), rather than that decade's biopics, in that it charts an individual's trip from a world of relative comfort and innocence to one of harsh reality. There is not much personal suffering for Guevara in *The Motorcycle Diaries* (unlike the hero in *I Am a Fugitive from a Chain Gang*), but witnessing the suffering of others lights the fire of his political awakening and activism.

The caveats about *Breast Men* and *The Motorcycle Diaries* can be dispensed with for *Kinsey* (2004), a four-square biopic that follows Alfred Kinsey's life from boyhood to old age (although not death).[44] Dr Kinsey was, like Pasteur, a natural scientist with a PhD rather than a medical doctor; but his work was unquestionably in the field of public health, if that specialty includes mental well-being. He laboured to enlighten the population about the diversity of (the mechanics of) sexual behaviour so as to offset the misery and guilt that ignorance engendered. The film ticks almost all of the boxes set out by Babington and Elena, and even features a classic montage sequence that depicts the accumulation of data, here neatly conveyed by interviewers' faces being progressively superimposed on a map of America (in *Dr Ehrlich's Magic Bullet*, it was a succession of the numbers of experiments conducted to find the magic bullet). As per the norm, the film was made roughly 50 years after the actual events that it depicts. However, here there is a twist. The director Bill Condon has admitted that one of his reasons for making the film was to defend the advances that Kinsey had pioneered (the 'ameliorated conditions' mentioned earlier) in the face of what he perceived to be an increasingly illiberal contemporary cultural tide (Grundmann, 2005). Science itself is rehabilitated, too (at least in relation to *Breast Men*), with Condon stating

---

44 Which is not to say that the film includes no concessions to modernity – for instance, the personal life of the hero is given increased attention, compared with the old films; and so is the role of Mrs Kinsey, the woman behind the man.

that 'Science is definitely the warm spot of the movie – the place where truth resides' (Grundmann, 2005, p. 11).

I hope it is apparent that genres are made up of a critical mass of films that are affiliated rather than identical to one another. The defined components of the genre may not exactly match any given film, but those films that hit eight or nine out of ten of them might be thought of as blood relations. We must allow that genres may evolve over time, too, as they are cumulative in nature, and influenced by their cultural context. In consequence, the concept of genre is useful as a heuristic device – by looking at films through the filter of genre, it can help us to see what is the same and what is different about things that are part of a tradition or set, and so to gauge how our expectations are (or are not) being met.

Genres have another function, too. They are a manifestation of 'the human need for archetypes and rituals' (Corrigan and White, 2004, p. 288), their central attraction lying in the very ingredients that have been often seen. From this it follows that in identifying a medical biopic genre, we gain a rich insight into what underpins the public perception of (medical-researcher-type) doctors.[45] Judging by *Kinsey*, this perception has not changed all that much in 70 years.

From there, it is only a small step to a recent paper by Schryer and Spoel (2005), in which they apply genre theory to case presentations and policy documents in the health field. They posit, among other things, that the set format of case presentations encourages medical students to move away from the use of (the patient's) lay language in describing illness symptoms towards the medical systems of thought embodied in professional terminology; and at the same time to take on, in less formal ways, the collegiate nature of their profession (for instance, via consultants' corrections of students in the form of 'We don't use that term, we say *x*'). Thus, they argue, the genre of case presentations is an influential element in the process of professional identity formation – that is, it provides a weighty contextual framework that, implicitly as well as explicitly, shapes the development and practice of health professionals. Genres, in other words, may not only shape public perceptions of the medical profession, but medical perceptions of it, too! Case

---

45 The fact that the films are accounts of 'historical fact' lends them even more popular credibility in this regard, albeit this is a somewhat spurious fillip, given the adjustments to the truth that are made in the films in the name of dramatic licence.

presentations, like biopics, are based on true stories, but plainly they only represent one particular version of that 'true story.' Maybe it behoves us all, then – patients, public, health professionals and all points in between – to be aware of the formulae by which real-life medical stories are passed around (in cinemas and on ward rounds); and to treasure films like *The Great Moment* which break out of the conventions without destroying them, thus reminding us that there are always alternatives.

References

Babington B. To catch a star on your fingertips: diagnosing the medical biopic from *The Story of Louis Pasteur* to *Freud*. In: Harper G, Moor A (eds) *Signs of Life: medicine and cinema*. London: Wallflower Press; 2005.

Corrigan T, White P. Rituals, conventions, archetypes and formulas: movie genres. In: *The Film Experience*. Boston, MA: Bedford/St Martin's; 2004.

Elena A. Exemplary lives: biographies of scientists on the screen. *Public Underst Sci.* 1993; **2**: 205–23.

Grundmann R. Too darn hot: Kinsey and the culture wars. *Cinéaste.* 2005; **30**: 4–10.

Schryer CF, Spoel P. Genre theory, health-care discourse, and professional identity formation. *J Bus Tech Commun.* 2005; **19**: 249–78.

Filmography

DR EHRLICH'S MAGIC BULLET (1940)

Credits

Director	William Dieterle
Producer	Hal B Wallis
Production Company	Warner Bros
Screenplay	John Huston, Heinz Herald, Norman Burnside
Music	Max Steiner
Photography	James Wong Howe
Editor	Warren Low
Art Director	Carl Jules Weyl

Cast

Dr Paul Ehrlich	Edward G Robinson
Hedwig Ehrlich	Ruth Gordon
Dr Emil von Behring	Otto Kruger
Dr Hans Wolfert	Sig Ruman

THE GREAT MOMENT (1944)

Credits

Director	Preston Sturges
Producer	BG De Sylva
Production Company	Paramount
Screenplay	Preston Sturges
Original book	Rene Fulop-Miller
Photography	Victor Milner
Editor	Stuart Gilmore
Art Director	Hans Dreier
Musical score	Victor Young

Cast

Dr Willam Morton	Joel McCrea
Elizabeth Morton	Betty Field
Professor Warren	Harry Carey
Eben Frost	William Demarest
Dr Jackson	Julian Tannen

BREAST MEN (1997)

Credits

Director	Lawrence O'Neill
Producer	Gary Lucchesi
Production Company	HBO
Screenplay	John Stockwell
Photography	Robert Stevens
Editor	Michael Jablow
Art Director	Jane Ann Stewart
Music	Dennis McCarthy

Cast

Dr Kevin Saunders	David Schwimmer
Dr William Larson	Chris Cooper

KINSEY (2004)

Credits

Director	Bill Condon
Producer	Gail Mutrux
Production Company	N1 European Film Produktions GmbH/ Zoetrope
Screenplay	Bill Condon
Photography	Frederick Elmes

Editor	Virginia Katz
Art Director	Nicholas Lundy
Music	Carter Burwell

Cast

Dr Alfred Kinsey	Liam Neeson
Clara McMillen	Laura Linney
Herman Wells	Oliver Platt
Thurman Rice	Tim Curry

THE MOTORCYCLE DIARIES (2004)

Credits

Director	Walter Salles
Producers	Michael Nozik, Edgard Tenembaum, Karen Tenkhoff
Production Companies	FilmFour, South Fork Pictures
Executive Producers	Robert Redford, Paul Webster, Rebecca Yeldham
Screenplay	José Rivera based on the books *The Motorcycle Diaries* by Ernesto Che Guevara and *With Che Through Latin America* by Alberto Granado
Photography	Éric Gautier
Editor	Daniel Rezende
Production Designer	Carlos Conti
Music	Gustavo Santaoalalla

Cast

Ernesto Guevara de la Serna	Gael García Bernal
Alberto Granado	Rodrigo de la Serna
Chichina	Mía Maestro
Celia de la Serna	Mercedes Moran
Dr Hugo Pesce	Gustavo Bueno
Dr Bresciani	Jorge Chiarella

CHAPTER 11

Great directors. II: Akira Kurosawa (1910–1998)

By 1951, Japanese cinema had a considerable history, the country having enthusiastically embraced the medium early in the twentieth century. However, the Western world was largely unaware of its existence until a film called *Rashomon* won top prize in the Venice Film Festival of that year, as well as winning a special Oscar for best foreign language film – in the process announcing the film's director, Akira Kurosawa, as one of the great artists of the cinema.

For the non-expert Westerner, watching Japanese films can involve a complicated cultural negotiation, and trying to read the mores and moods of a country with very different characteristics might appear a daunting task. In the cinema, for instance, kissing on screen was unheard of before the Second World War; and what are we to make of what Richie has called a 'notorious predilection for the unhappy ending' (Richie, 1982, p. 42)? Plainly, an unthinking imposition of Western values would be rash. And yet the immediate post-war period was, for obvious reasons, a time of great reassessment and change in Japan, and maybe these circumstances contributed to making the country's films more accessible to foreigners. That said, the truth is probably that directors of the stature of Kurosawa (or some of his slightly older peers, such as Ozu and Naruse) explore themes so profound that they are universally understandable, and timeless.[46] Certainly Kurosawa is such

---

46 Interestingly, there has been a two-way cultural exchange with Kurosawa. He has made wonderful film versions of Shakespeare (*Throne of Blood* is arguably the greatest filmed 'Macbeth'); and has himself been adapted by Western film-makers – most

a fantastic storyteller, and a cinematographer of such dynamism, that his films brush past the trepidation of most newcomers like a president walking through passport control.

His three doctor movies are – regardless of our special interest in this book – superb films, especially the first and last. All of them offer major meditations on life in general, as well as on specific different facets of what it means to be a doctor. They are not a series in any sequential sense – they feature very different doctors and tell very different stories – so it doesn't really matter which of the films you watch first.

Drunken Angel (1948)

One might describe the first scene of this film as an absolute knockout, but that would imply finality when it is very much a beginning. The camera roves around a slum district late at night before settling inside an empty, darkened room. A middle-aged man comes in, bringing some light with him from the corridor outside, and we see that the room is no better appointed than the neighbourhood in which it is located. The man switches on the light and starts half-heartedly flicking dust off the furnishings with a cloth. He is dishevelled, with a four-day beard, a toothpick and an air of having gone to seed; but we notice that he is a doctor (because of his white coat, unbuttoned due to the heat and with no shirt underneath) and that this is a consulting room (because of the instruments on the desk). He is followed in by a patient with a damaged hand, who has apparently come to see him in the middle of the night for urgent help. The patient is younger than the doctor and better groomed, his hair is parted and combed back, his clothes are stylish in a flashy kind of way; and he is undoubtedly good-looking. The doctor takes little interest in his patient, barely looking at him for much of the consultation, and going about his work on apparent autopilot. By contrast, at one point he tries to leave the door open to create a draught, only to find that it keeps closing, whereupon he becomes extremely engaged. He hunkers down to study the door closely; examines the hinges; and mulls over possible solutions; before reaching for a bin to prop it open – all this while the patient sits waiting for treatment!

The patient has a hand injury that he claims was caused by shutting it in a door. The doctor does not contradict him as he examines the hand, and merely

famously, *The Magnificent Seven* (Sturges, 1960) was a remake of Kurosawa's *Seven Samurai* (1954).

says 'I suppose you call this a nail' as he extracts a bullet. The young man, who is named Matsunaga, is unembarrassed about his lie, and says that he was a participant in 'just a little fight.' Opening up the flesh of the palm with clamps, the doctor proceeds to clean out the wound, heedless of the agony he is causing the patient, who struggles to maintain his unflinching front – as indeed do we the audience! Instead, he tells him (when it is too late for the patient to opt out) 'I warn you my fees are very high – I always overcharge people who eat and drink too much', thereby revealing the moral judgement that he has made. Given his own somewhat shabby condition, and his apparent apathy, this stance comes as a slight surprise to us.

The patient's hand now properly dressed, the consultation is apparently over when the patient's cough attracts attention. 'People like you are susceptible to tuberculosis', says the doctor. 'Me? With a body like this?' retorts Matsunaga, his cool recovered now that the minor surgery is over. 'You can't go by appearances' says the doctor, bringing one of the subtexts of the scene closer to the surface. 'You'll just have a cough and won't feel any pain. By the time you realise you've got it, it's too late. Are you scared?' At this point Kurosawa cuts to the first close-up of the film, as Matsunaga's face attempts to conceal his alarm. 'Scared?' he says, and flicking his cigarette at the doctor he continues 'Don't play the high and mighty with me. You're just trying to make money.' He throws his jacket down like a gauntlet and says 'Go on, then – tell me if I've got TB', and sits back down in the patient's seat – which suggests that he is indeed scared of the disease. The doctor does not rise to this challenge to his manhood (routed through his professionalism), and replies 'How do you suppose I do that? Do you think I can diagnose TB just by tapping your chest, listening with my stethoscope, and cocking my head?', all of which he proceeds to do, including making the diagnosis. This we see on his face in *his* first close-up, as he holds a stethoscope to Matsunaga's back. His proficiency is further proof of his continued clinical competence, notwithstanding his reduced circumstances. As he washes his hands, he tells Matsunaga in a matter-of-fact way to get himself X-rayed; and that he might not have long to live. Immediately, Matsunaga becomes enraged, evidently blaming the messenger. With his good hand he grabs the doctor by the scruff of the neck and pins him down on the examining table, shouting at him. The doctor does not mount any resistance. Only when a nurse makes a belated entry is the situation defused. Matsunaga re-dons his protective swagger as he walks out of the room, while the doctor, in his own belated fit of fury, throws a cushion at the departing man's head. When the young man has gone, Sanada says to the nurse 'Thugs like him just laugh at TB. But he can still make me worry about him, so he must have a bit of humanity left . . .'

It is a long, unhurried opening scene (lasting over 7 minutes) and a brilliant start to a film, laden with atmosphere and subtle exposition of character, yet seeming entirely natural. It sets up the central driver of the film – the symbiotic love–hate relationship between Sanada the doctor and Matsunaga the gangster, which grows out of the love–hate relationship that they seem to have with themselves. Sanada is plainly a good man – intelligent, principled and kindly – who has let himself be bested by life and is now cantankerous and curmudgeonly. We are not spared sight of his unheroic behaviour – he is frequently thrown out of places for being a nuisance, and he is needlessly rude to people, often because of his alcohol intake (hence the film's title). Matsunaga meets him going in the opposite direction, a petty crook and bully who aspires to nobility. He believes in, and lives by, a code of honour (which none of his fellow gangsters do), subscribing to a romantic myth of his role in a way that the doctor has long since abandoned. Matsunaga's aspirations lead to his downfall, but also to Sanada trying to save him, as noted in the first scene. Through this process, both men touch their repressed humanity, although it can hardly be said that they change their spots – the film is too unsentimental for that. However, the story does not have one of the unhappy endings that Richie (1984) refers to. While Matsunaga is ultimately imprisoned by his past, another of Sanada's patients, a young girl who also has TB, is cured at the end of the film. And the message about the doctor himself appears to be that a drunken angel is the right man in the right place for the job, precisely because he is a fully paid up member of the flawed community that he serves,[47] rather than a knight on a white charger.

The Quiet Duel (1949)

Whereas *Drunken Angel* is built around a complex doctor–patient relationship, *The Quiet Duel* is primarily concerned with a doctor's internal struggle (which is why the duel is quiet). However, although it is not about relationships (in the intimate sense), one of its key themes is how people affect one another.

Kyoji, a young male doctor, exhausted and working in atrocious conditions in a military field hospital at the end of World War Two, removes his

---

47 The story's backdrop of post-war urban Japan is worthy of a book chapter in itself, as tradition rubs shoulders uncomfortably with new elements that reflect the (unseen) American conquerors.

surgical gloves because they are slowing him down during a time-pressured operation. He then nicks his finger on a scalpel; and the theoretical possibility of cross-infection proves to be all too real when blood tests a few days later show that he has contracted syphilis.

After the war, he works with his father in a small community maternity hospital, but shies away from his fiancée Misao. We the audience know that this is because of his disease, but no one else is party to this information until a nurse walks in on Kyoji injecting himself with Salvarsan (as invented by Dr Ehrlich in the preceding chapter of this book!). Kyoji's reasoning is that Misao is such a good woman that she would wait for the many years it will take to effect his cure, even at the risk of losing the opportunity to have children. Kyoji loves her too much to want her to suffer for him, so he does all he can to sever relations with her without telling her why.[48] He also fears that people will not believe that he did not catch syphilis in the more usual way (i.e. through sex and, by extension, loose morals). Misao eventually takes the hint and, heartbroken, marries someone else.

Kyoji happens upon Nakada, the man who 'gave' him his disease, and makes strenuous efforts – which are ultimately unsuccessful – to persuade him to seek a cure before he ruins his own health as well as that of his wife (and unborn baby). The film ends with Nakada's wife recovering in the community hospital after a stillbirth.

As per the film's title, Kyoji's duel is the central plank of the narrative. In part, it is a duel with his disease; but more importantly, his struggle is to maintain a code of conduct in the face of tribulation. This code of conduct is tied up with being a doctor in his eyes. At one point he tells a patient, 'You have to think about other people's happiness rather than your own', and this is clearly the principle by which he lives. To accomplish this, he adopts a buttoned-up outward persona throughout, summed up in the following exchange with the nurse:

> Kyoji: 'There are two kinds of patient: some scream in pain, others put up with pain dripping with sweat.'
>
> Nurse Minegishi: 'And you're the dripping with sweat kind?'
>
> Kyoji: 'Because I don't like losing . . . and I am a doctor.'

---

48 This may be a sticking point in the film for viewers today, who may feel that the set-up is being milked a little to generate pathos.

Kyoji has just seen his ex-fiancée, and she has told him that she is getting married the next day. When she has left, Kyoji breaks down in front of Minegishi, succumbing for the one and only time to self-pity ('Why do I have to suffer so much?'). He bares his soul and is in tears, confessing to the agonising frustration of self-denial. Only when Minegishi also breaks down in tears at his plight does he pull himself together. And the symbol of his recomposure is his stethoscope, shown in close-up as Kyoji picks it up and heads off back to work.

Nurse Minegishi's tears are a symbol, too. She had started the film as an assistant nurse, depressed to the point of being suicidal because she was pregnant but unmarried ('Poor people should die early for their own good'). When she walks in on Kyoji injecting himself, she experiences a certain *Schadenfreude*, assuming that she has uncovered moral hypocrisy. It is only when she overhears him explaining the true cause of his disease to his father that she appreciates the unhappiness of others, and this is the catalyst for her own transformation into someone who not only takes responsibility for herself, but also cares for other people. Entirely unwittingly, Kyoji has acted as a role model, and he continues to inspire her (and others) for the rest of the film. As modern-day viewers, we may not entirely agree with Kyoji's great self-expectations; but many of us will surely recognise the romantic attraction of his paragon-of-virtue philosophy and consequent behaviour. A local policeman who has flitted in and out of the film says that Kyoji is 'a saint amongst doctors', to which Kyoji's father replies, 'He's just trying to give hope back to people who are unhappier than he is. If he had been happy, he might have become a snob.' The film helps its case no end by eschewing easy sentiment, the ending supplying little in the way of the usual closure. Kyoji and his fiancée are not reunited, and she is apprised at last of the truth; Minegishi, despite reconstructing herself, does not have an amorous relationship with Kyoji (notwithstanding the fact that she is in love with him); and nor does he conveniently 'discover' a love for her as a substitute for Misao. Kyoji is not cured of his syphilis (although it is apparently well controlled). The last shot of the film simply shows Kyoji and his father and Nurse Minegishi working together closely as a team, performing an operation.

Red Beard (1965)

Having suggested earlier that the order in which you see the films in this chapter does not matter, there is perhaps a case for watching this one last. This is not because it is the most recent, or the most pertinent; but merely because the doctor in this film has a degree of maturity and self-knowledge that the protagonists (medical or otherwise) in the other films do not possess, so it makes a logical final instalment. The effect is increased by the fact that the main doctor is played by the great Toshiro Mifune (who acted as the gangster in *Drunken Angel* and the doctor in *The Quiet Duel*), and he is now more than 15 years older, of course.[49]

Mifune plays the part of Dr Niide, known as Red Beard, and he dominates the film, although this is as much through sheer force of personality as share of screen time. Paradoxically, plenty of space is accorded to patients' stories, because this mirrors Niide's philosophy. At one point he explains to his trainee Yasumoto[50] that 'Behind every illness there is always a story of misfortune.'

Red Beard's approach is unconventional, both in theory and in deed. He is a sensitive, caring man who practises tough love and is unafraid to bloody a few noses (literally) if needs must. Often the harsh conditions of the clinic that he runs are due to shortage of funds, but he turns the enforced ascetic lifestyle into a basis for clinical and moral gain. For example, the patients' sleeping mats are thin because they are more hygienic; and the doctors' basic uniforms allow the local community to recognise them as clinic (i.e. free) doctors and make them approachable. Yasumoto, already angry about his indenture because he has aspirations to work for the shogunate, is unhappy about the quality of the meals served to the staff, and is told by Red Beard that 'Even bad food tastes good if you chew it well. It's the same with our work.'

This existential bent allows Red Beard to simultaneously embody self-confidence and humility. At one point, Yasumoto asks him about a particular patient: 'There's no cure?' Red Beard replies 'No – but not only for this case. There are no cures really. . . . Medical science doesn't know anything. We recognise symptoms, developments, we try to help. But that's about all. We can only fight poverty and ignorance; and mask our own ignorance.'

However, his philosophical stance does not preclude direct action, and he is nothing if not pragmatic. Apart from his numerous clinical interventions with patients, he also knows how to be a fixer, at one point leaning on a local magistrate to waive charges against a female patient who has, in extreme mitigating circumstances, committed and confessed to a crime. (This episode

---

49 Coincidentally, *Red Beard* was the final collaboration between Mifune and Kurosawa, and *Drunken Angel* had been the first. In between, the two men were one of the great partnerships of cinema history.

50 Yasumoto is in fact the hook for the storyline, such as it is. The film is 'about' his period of apprenticeship with Red Beard.

again shows his humility. Red Beard is ashamed because he has threatened the magistrate by hints rather than open statement. 'If ever I'm arrogant, remind me of today', he says to Yasumoto, and this is the only time in the film when his eyes are shifty.)

The most memorable instance of direct action occurs in a scene where Red Beard and Yasumoto go to the local brothel to check on the prostitutes' health. There, Red Beard is displeased to find a 13-year-old girl whom the madame wants to press into service. He insists on taking her away with him, and is faced by a gang of the madame's enforcers. In a wonderful fight sequence, he sees them all off with an effortless demonstration of martial art – an extraordinary flourish in an otherwise reflective and thoughtful film! We see (and hear) him breaking bones with complete ruthlessness, although he expresses compunction afterwards. 'Such violence is awful', he says as he puts back someone's jaw which he has just dislocated. 'A doctor should not do such things. I may have gone too far – I was too heavy-handed.'

Even in the heat of this battle, there is no sense that he is losing his temper, and this calm characterises all of his encounters, whether with enemies, patients or junior colleagues. The young girl, now safely ensconced back in the clinic, falls sick but refuses all medicine. Red Beard comes to try to administer her syrup, but she repeatedly knocks the spoon away as he holds it out to her. Yet he persists patiently, realising that too many people have been angry with her in the past for that response to serve any useful purpose. Similarly, when Yasumoto makes a grave error of professional judgement which nearly costs him his life, Red Beard simply says 'Don't be ashamed, but let it be a lesson to you.'

As may be becoming evident, *Red Beard* is almost inspirational in nature. Here we have a doctor who understands that the practice of medicine involves mixing science with social awareness and psychological insight (not to mention a teaching component), and who delivers on every front. The narrative ingredients of Yasumoto's apprenticeship are simple and well rehearsed in many other medical films; yet here simplicity translates into nobility, whereas so often it signals a descent into banality. At nearly three hours, the running time of the film may be a deterrent, as might its period setting; but it is not at all arduous to watch, and its unhurried style seems completely normal once one is immersed in it.

Watching all of these Kurosawa films, you cannot help feeling that you are in the presence of a master as, apparently effortlessly, he fuses implacable wisdom with technical brilliance. He was one of the founding fathers of humanist cinema, along with people like Jean Renoir, Vittorio de Sica, Satyajit Ray and Ingmar Bergman – people who, when you see their films, make you think that *this* is what cinema should be. It is our good fortune that he put medicine at the centre of his stories on several occasions, and it is an honour to include him in this book.

References

Richie D. *The Japanese Movie*. Tokyo: Kodansha; 1982.
Richie D. *The Films of Akira Kurosawa*. Berkeley, CA: University of California Press; 1984.

Filmography

DRUNKEN ANGEL [YOIDORE TENSHI] (1948)

Credits

Director	Akira Kurosawa
Producers	Sojiro Motoki
Production Company	Toho
Screenplay	Keinosuki Uekusa, Akira Kurosawa
Photography	Takeo Ito
Editor	Akira Kurosawa
Art Director	So Matsuyama
Music	Fumio Hayasaka

Cast

Dr Sanada	Takashi Shimura
Matsunaga	Toshiro Mifune
Okada	Reisaburo Yamamoto
Nanae	Michiyo Kogure
Gin	Noriko Sengoku

THE QUIET DUEL [SHIZUKANARU KETTO] (1949)

Credits

Director	Akira Kurosawa
Producers	Sojiro Motoki, Hisao Ichikawa
Production Company	Daiei
Screenplay	Senkichi Taniguchi, Akira Kurosawa
Original play	Kazuo Kikuta
Photography	Shoichi Aisaka
Editor	Masanori Tsujii

Art Director	Koichi Imai
Music	Akira Ifukube

Cast

Dr Kyoji Fujisaki	Toshiro Mifune
Dr Konosuke Fujisaki	Takashi Shimura
Misao Matsumoto	Miki Sanjo
Nurse Rui Minegishi	Noriko Sengoku
Susumu Nakada	Kenjiro Uemura
Takiko Nakada	Chieko Nakakita

RED BEARD [AKAHIGE] (1965)

Credits

Director	Akira Kurosawa
Producers	Ryuzo Kikushima, Tomoyuki Tanaka
Production Companies	Toho, Kurosawa Productions
Screenplay	Ryuzo Kikushima, Hdeo Oguni, Masato Ide, Akira Kurosawa
Original novel	Shugoro Yamamoto
Photography	Asakazu Nakai, Takuo Saito
Editor	Reiko Kaneko
Art Director	Yoshiro Muraki
Music	Masaru Sato

Cast

Dr Kyojio Niide, 'Red Beard'	Toshiro Mifune
Dr Noboru Yasumoto	Yuzo Kyama
Dr Handayu Mori	Yoshio Tsuchiya
Genzo Tsugawa	Tatsuyoshi Ehara
Osui	Reiko Dan
Mad woman	Kyoko Kagawa
Tokubei Izumiya	Takashi Shimura

CHAPTER 12

Doctors, in practice

One way of learning about the characteristics of a profession is to watch some-one doing an impersonation of one of its members. If you wanted to pretend to be a doctor, how would you act? We shall start this chapter by running the rule over a couple of films that feature ersatz medics, before moving on to two that put 'real' medical practice at the centre of their stories.[51]

Meet the fakers

An anxious young woman wanders along a corridor in a typical old-style office building, in search of the room for her private appointment with Dr Monnier. Seeing a man backing out of a door saying that he will be back next week, she walks past him into the antechamber of what she takes to be a psychoanalyst's consulting rooms. A conservatively dressed man gestures her through to the inner sanctum in which a *fin de siècle* couch is prominently positioned, as he finishes off a call about another client who is evidently in the midst of a personal crisis. The woman settles herself down in a chair and promptly starts to unburden herself about her marital difficulties, blurting out many details in her obvious distress. The only problem is that the man she is talking to is an accountant, and the couch is there for his afternoon naps – she has stepped into the wrong office. The initial mistaken identity is plausible (there are several visual and verbal cues that apparently reinforce the woman's assumption) and it is mutual. When she launches into her tale of woe, the accountant, taking it to be a prelude to some divorce settlement discussion, makes encouraging noises (including using the open question-ing that is emphasised in medical school communication skills courses), and

---

51 Of course, both types of film are fictions . . .

gets ready to take notes,[52] shrink-like. It is only after a few minutes, when he realises that she is not going to get to the financial point, and indeed must be confusing his occupation, that he knowingly – albeit passively – prolongs the mix-up. She departs hastily, only pausing to confirm that he is willing to take her on as a patient. As we find out more about him in the next few minutes of the film, we can see why he might want to buy into such a hoax.

He fits most of the stereotypes associated with accountants: he is overly orderly, physically uninspiring and generally short of sparkle – one might say 'middle-aged', regardless of his date of birth. A divorcé who has a slightly masochistic relationship with his ex-wife, it is evident that turning into a psychoanalyst offers several immediate benefits. It gives him instant access to the intimate details of a young woman's life (her conjugal bed being a more interesting topic than a tax rebate); he is cast in the part of heroic rescuer (in effect, a jump up from his usual cameo role to top-billing); and he will be able to have more of the same on a weekly basis, in an unusual twist on the concept of continuity of care. In short, his new-found medical status seems to fix his twin life problems of being bored and boring.[53] It is made clear that these possibilities are all predicated on the patient being a good-looking woman. For instance, we see other clients who seem to use him for emotional as well as accountancy support, but he provides as little of this as he can get away with because they are not sexually attractive.

They get through one more session a week later, with the accountant making half-hearted (and unsuccessful) efforts to come clean; but this being a drama rather than a Hitchcockian thriller, it is not long before the woman discovers her error. She confronts him angrily, and he duly apologises. And then a curious thing happens: just as she is about to storm out of his office, she asks if they can continue with their weekly appointments. At this point the question shifts to why she should do this, knowing that he is not a doctor;[54] and the film turns into a study of a relationship between two particular people, rather than a commentary on doctors and patients in general. (It is worth watching, and is called *Confidences Trop Intimes* (2004, Leconte). The English title is *Intimate Strangers*, which is not quite the same thing.)

---

52 The point that it is not only doctors who are given privileged access to people's private lives, and who serve a Wailing-Wall function, is well made.

53 The realisation of this truth prompts the accountant to become a patient of the real Dr Monnier further down the corridor.

54 Indeed, a separate chapter (in a separate book) could be written about projection on the part of patients and even communities.

As already noted, the start of that film operates a little like one of Hitchcock's 'wrong man' movies, where a protagonist is propelled into a radically different world on the basis of being mistaken for someone else. *Paper Mask* (1991, Morahan) works on the opposite premise – the central character is continually presumed innocent when in fact he is thoroughly guilty. (Perhaps Patricia Highsmith's character Thomas Ripley is the relevant cultural reference in this case.)

Written by John Collee, a doctor-turned-writer, this film *is* a thriller of sorts, in which the protracted role playing of the main character – a young porter-turned-doctor – is rooted in some fairly serious psychopathy. Assuming the identity of a medic whom he has seen killed in a road accident, hospital auxiliary Matthew Harris proceeds to grow into the part of a jobbing junior doctor. Initially armed only with a smattering of clinical knowledge and a good understanding of the day-to-day workings of a hospital (both picked up by close observation), he assiduously mugs up textbooks, and cleverly moves about from one organisational blind spot to another, and gets by, frequently by the skin of his teeth. Thanks to Collee's background, the film convincingly presents several scenes in which Harris's pretence is entirely believable. For instance, when confronted by an illuminated X-ray that he is at a loss to interpret, he light-heartedly bets a colleague standing next to him ten pence that she cannot name the diagnosis. She proudly proceeds to do so, thus educating him for a very small tuition fee! Perhaps the most alarming section of the film – for the audience, at least – is his first day in a casualty job, where his utter incompetence is regarded as normal by a Sister who has seen too many new doctors fresh out of medical school to be even mildly surprised. Indeed, by taking him under her wing, she facilitates this rake's progress.

Notwithstanding his skill as a conman, the film demonstrates how the world turns on an axis of trust. Someone who is wearing a white coat in a hospital and intimating that they are a doctor must *ipso facto* be one; and considerable allowances will be made before there is a paradigm shift to doubt and suspicion. In part, Harris is the method actor who ends up believing in his own act, not least because he is enjoying the quantum leap in social status of his new role and the attendant gains (as in *Confidences Trop Intimes*, increased sexual allure features among these); but there is also a large element of self-preservation involved, as the only way for him to avoid recriminations is to plunge ever deeper into his fabrication. His special talent is to judge nicely when to own up to his ignorance – a trait that is seen as endearingly honest by nurses – and when to cover up and play for time (in front of consultants). It would seem here that manners plus motivation maketh man.

A litany of ills, and some remedies

These tales of imposture may serve to make us aware, *en passant*, of certain aspects of being a doctor – the performance component and the aura that surrounds the profession, in particular. However, the next two films mount a broadside on medicine, and are explicitly designed to give a wide-ranging appraisal of its possibilities and problem areas.

Not surprisingly, given its to-the-point title, *The Doctor* (1991, Haines)[55] has plenty to say about medical practice. Discussing it after a screening with some GPs, I suggested that the screenplay must have been written by a medical sociologist, so zealously did it draw together many of the main strands of criticism of modern medicine. Later on, to substantiate my claim (although no one seemed to disagree with me), I looked up the contemporaneous edition of *Sociology as Applied to Medicine* (Scambler, 1991), the widely used textbook for medical students, and set about trying to cross-match boxes. Since the film is American and the book British, there is inevitably a little disparity in the detail; but taken overall, the shared interests abound, and are as follows:

'Chapter 3 – Health and illness behaviour': This chapter reviews lay beliefs about health and illness and how they influence the use of health services. In the film, there are two prominent patients whose health and illness behaviour are especially pertinent. The eponymous doctor, Jack McKee, ignores his own symptoms (a recurrent cough) until they reach a trigger point (in terms of severity) when he finds blood on his handkerchief. Up until then he had been a fully paid up H_2O molecule in the clinical iceberg.[56] His propensity for denial is a good fit with his character; and his acceptance of sickness is the start of the journey to personal and professional redemption that is the story's core. Then, near the end of the film, McKee treats a Latin American transplant patient who has concerns about the metaphysical aspects of organ donation that need to be addressed before he will proceed. The new improved McKee works through the worries of the patient and his family sensitively, and so clears the obstruction to the patient's survival.

'Chapter 4 – The doctor–patient relationship': There is an emphatic tick next to this one, as already noted in (this book's) Chapter 5. We witness power

55 As seen in Chapter 5.
56 This neatly makes the point that doctors are lay people, too!

struggles between patients and doctors (McKee and his doctors); communication breakdown leading to patient dissatisfaction (McKee and his female surgeon); different consulting styles (McKee and his family practitioner); and so on. Incidentally, Lucy Fischer has written a helpful piece purely on the subject of empathy in the film (Fischer, 2004).

'Chapter 5 – 'Hospitals and patients': There are several scenes that illustrate the chapter's assertions about hospitals being simultaneously formal and informal organisations. The film shows traditional hierarchies being observed (e.g. patients and staff deferring to consultants), as well as instances where matters of import are decided according to personal preference in private conversations (e.g. McKee withdrawing support for a colleague in a litigation case).

And so we can go on, through Chapter 6 ('Living with chronic illness'), Chapter 7 ('Dying, death and bereavement'), Chapter 9 ('Women as patients and providers'), Chapter 12 ('The limits of medical knowledge'), Chapter 13 ('Deviance, sick role and stigma') and Chapter 15 ('Health professions'). The book has 19 chapters, and the subjects of nine of them (i.e. nearly half) are addressed in *The Doctor*. Although the film is by no means entirely critical, it nonetheless amounts to a serious indictment of medicine in 1991 – most centrally, that its charge towards technical proficiency (not to mention commercial viability) causes the collateral damage of emotional illiteracy in its practitioners.

It is sad but perhaps not all together surprising that deficiencies highlighted in 1991 have yet to be eradicated. However, it is downright disheartening that a film made about medicine 40 years *before that* is still highly pertinent. *People Will Talk* (1951, Mankiewicz), which has a somewhat ambiguous and (misleadingly) flippant-sounding title, appears to be another example of how human knowledge outstrips the ability to implement it; and how Art often says things before academia (even social science!).

The film opens with three intertitles, superimposed on images of an august seat of learning, that are a declaration of intent: 'This will be part of the story of Noah Praetorius, MD. That is not his real name of course . . . /There may be some who will claim to identify Dr Praetorius at once. There may be some who will reject the possibility that such a doctor lives, or could have lived. And there will be some who will hope that if he hasn't, or doesn't, he most certainly should . . . /Our story is also – always with high regard – about Medicine and the Medical Profession. Respectfully, therefore, with humble gratitude, this film is dedicated to one who has inspired man's unending battle

against Death, and without whom that battle is never won . . . the patient.'
If the meaning of the first two pronouncements is a little cryptic at this stage
of the proceedings, the third nails the film's colours to the mast – patients are
the horse to the doctors' cart.

The film's overarching storyline concerns the efforts of a colleague to
ground the aforementioned high-flying Dr Praetorius by bringing to bear
charges of misconduct against him. This attempt is shown to be baseless
and vindictive, and so portrays the internal affairs of the medical profession
in a bad light – quite apart from the obvious echo it provides of the anti-
communist 'witch-hunt' being prosecuted at that time in America.

During the course of the film a barrage of criticism (albeit calm and articulate) is aimed at modern medicine. The first shot is fired in the first scene, when
a layperson says to the villain of the piece, 'You're a professor, and it's hard
to make you understand anything that ain't in a book. Most of what goes on
in the world ain't in a book.' Meanwhile our first exposure to Praetorius[57]
finds him waiting in a lecture theatre full of medical students, whereupon
he embarks on an impromptu exploration of Cartesian duality, only to be
interrupted by a plot point from the film's second storyline. (Although this
latter storyline notionally centres on romance, it is also an important vehicle
for other issues, as we shall see.) Later, the film trains its sights on (among
other things) the importance of hospital architecture; the need to build systems around patients, not staff or simplistic budgetary considerations ('Bad
therapy is never good economy'); and the clear-sightedness required to define
medicine's mission statement. Praetorius challenges a scientist friend who is
suggesting that patients' emotional lives are none of his business. He asks
'What *is* my business?', to which his friend replies, 'To diagnose the physical
ails of human beings and to cure them.' Praetorius responds 'Wrong. My business is to make sick people well – there's a vast difference.' To this end, he has
set up his own clinic-cum-hospital (a polyclinic, perhaps, except that it concentrates on women's health) where things can be run according to 'my belief
that patients are sick people, not inmates.' However, even here Praetorius has
to work hard to change norms. At one point he upbraids his nurses for der-
eliction of duty, when their habitual inattentiveness puts a patient at risk. A
previous attempt to create an environment in which he could practise medicine as he envisaged it saw Praetorius take the unusual step of setting up shop

---

57 Played by Cary Grant, in the third of his three fascinating medical films (see also
  Chapter 4, and *Every Girl Should Be Married* (1948, Hartman)).

(literally) as a butcher in a small rural town. Under the disarming cover of selling meat ('at cost'!), he could integrate himself into the community, and was able to dispense a variety of treatments (whether pills, scalpels or 'sometimes just talking a body into being well'), to the immense gratitude of the locals. (It is evident from the few consultations we observe that Praetorius has an easy way with people that pushes the doctor–patient relationship towards equality and away from the traditional *de haut en bas* model.)

Aside from his independent views on an alarmingly contemporarily relevant variety of societal ills (he is anti-creationism, anti-nuclear and anti-farm subsidies, but pro-farm shops), Praetorius' non-conformism extends to his views on sexual morality. In the story strand that encompasses romance, he makes no moral judgement on a single woman who is pregnant; and indeed upon discovering that he is in love with her, he has no qualms about proposing marriage in the knowledge that he will be the (legal) father of another man's (biological) child.

There are some ingredients of the film that will sit uneasily with modern audiences, and it is evidently the product of a particular brand of post-war liberal sensibility, but both its trenchant critique and its enlightened alternative remain apropos. Nobody ever said that the practice of medicine was simple, although sometimes one gets the impression that nobody ever said that it wasn't either, judging by the over-confidence of some of its practitioners. Cinema is one way in which society gets to express its displeasure with these would-be supremos. Praetorius is a doctor who understands his role in the world, and has neither too high nor too low an opinion of himself. He is no less fictional than the pretenders with which we started the chapter. However, if the character of Matthew Harris in *Paper Mask* highlights certain societal anxieties about the power of the mantle of medicine, then Noah Praetorius perhaps represents some of our belief that things can get better. As one of the intertitles at the start of the film states: 'There may be some who will reject the possibility that such a doctor lives, or could have lived. And there will be some who will hope that if he hasn't, or doesn't, he most certainly should . . .'

References

Fischer L. Big boys do cry: empathy in *The Doctor*. In: *Cultural Sutures: medicine and media*. Durham, NC: Duke University Press; 2004.

Scambler G (ed.) *Sociology as Applied to Medicine*. 3rd ed. London: Baillière Tindall; 1991.

Filmography

CONFIDENCES TROP INTIMES (2004)

Credits

Director	Patrice Leconte
Production Companies	France 3 Cinéma, Canal+
Executive Producer	Christine Gozlan
Producer/Presenter	Jérôme Sarde
Scénario/Dialogue	Jérôme Tonnerre
Adaptation	Patrice Leconte
Photography Director	Eduardo Serra
Editing	Joëlle Hache
Art Director	Ivan Maussion
Composer of original music	Pascale Esteve

Cast

Anna	Sandrine Bonnaire
William	Fabrice Luchini
Doctor Monnier	Michel Duchaussoy

PAPER MASK (1991)

Credits

Director	Christopher Morahan
Production Company	Film Four International
Producer	Christopher Morahan
Screenplay	John Collee
Photography Director	Nat Crosby
Editor	Peter Coulson
Art Director	Andrew Rothschild
Music	Richard Harvey

Cast

Matthew Harris	Paul McGann
Christine Taylor	Amanda Donohoe
Dr Mumford	Frederick Treves
Dr Thorn	Tom Wilkinson
Celia Mumford	Barbara Leigh-Hunt
Alec Moran	Jimmy Yuill
Dr Lloyd	Mark Lewis Jones
Dr Hammond	John Warnaby

THE DOCTOR (1991)

Credits

Director	Randa Haines
Producer	Laura Ziskin
Production Company	Touchstone
Screenplay	Robert Caswell
Original story	Ed Rosenbaum
Photography	John Seale
Editor	Lisa Fruchtman
Art Director	Ken Adam
Music	Michael Convertino

Cast

Dr Jack McKee	William Hurt
Anne McKee	Christine Lahti
June Ellis	Elizabeth Perkins
Dr Murray Kaplan	Mandy Patinkin
Dr Eli Blumfield	Adam Arkin
Dr Lesley Abbott	Wendy Crewson

PEOPLE WILL TALK (1951)

Credits

Director	Joseph L Mankiewicz
Producer	Darryl F Zanuck
Production Company	Twentieth Century Fox
Screenplay	Joseph L Mankiewicz
Original play	Curt Goetz
Photography	Milton Krasner
Editor	Barbra McLean
Art Director	Lyle Wheeler

Cast

Dr Noah Praetorius	Cary Grant
Deborah Higgins	Jeanne Crain
Professor Elwell	Hume Cronyn
Shunderson	Finlay Currie
Professor Barker	Walter Slezak
Arthur Higgins	Sidney Blackmer

CHAPTER 13

Bigger than life? Medical melodrama

Melodrama is something of an ugly-duckling genre. Looked down on by men and women of 'good taste', it has been a beautiful swan – as indicated by cinema admissions – in the eyes of filmgoers and, consequently, the movie industry. In an intriguing twist, the pro-camp has been joined by the film studies critical fraternity/sorority in recent years.

The genre is a slippery customer to define. The etymology takes us back to certain theatre productions of the early nineteenth century that used music to bolster some scenes (*melos* – as in 'melody' – is Greek for music). So the first characteristic is perhaps the adoption of a strategy for heightening emotions – but then most films do that to a greater or lesser extent. Let us therefore put melodramas at the 'greater' end of that spectrum. Returning to music, whereas most classical compositions include some quiet passages, and a sense of counterbalance among the different sections of the orchestra, melodramas tend to have everyone playing *fortissimo* from start to finish. This can certainly make for a powerful experience in the front row of the stalls. Melodramas are often crammed with credibility-stretching incidents, which can take them somewhere beyond far-fetched. They are sometimes labelled 'women's pictures' – that is, pictures *for* women; but they are also frequently pictures *about* women, and strong women at that, and on that basis are an interesting phenomenon in the male-dominated oeuvre of mainstream cinema. German émigré Douglas Sirk was one of the most celebrated directors of classic Hollywood melodramas, and a commentator, writing about a female character in one of his films, talks of 'a typically resourceful but unhappy Sirkian heroine' (Finler, 1985) – an illuminating encapsulation.

Doctors are not infrequent participants in movie melodramas. It might be argued that they are usually only there contingently, because it is actually sickness that is the active story ingredient, as it has plenty of potential for heightening emotions. However, that line does not wholly meet the case in our first example (which was also Sirk's first big hit), where medicine is one operationalisation of the title.

Magnificent Obsession (Sirk, 1954)

The film tells the intertwining stories of Bob Merrick and Helen Phillips. Helen is married to Dr Wayne Phillips, a local hero in the small town of Brightwood where he runs a hospital. Considerably older than Helen, Dr Phillips suffers a heart attack; and dies because the resuscitator he requires is in use elsewhere at the critical moment. The resuscitator did indeed save a life – that of the local playboy son of a millionaire, who had crashed his powerboat while trying to break his own speed record just for the fun of it. This ne'er-do-well is Bob Merrick. To add to the already appreciable opprobrium headed in his direction, when Merrick is recuperating in Phillips' hospital he behaves with his usual graceless egocentricity, and even manages to pitch some crude chat-up lines at Helen Phillips (albeit when neither knows who the other is). He modifies his behaviour a little when he is informed of the repercussions of his irresponsibility, but the die is cast in Helen's mind, and that of her ally, Phillips' daughter Joyce. From this mildly bizarre situation there grows, perhaps predictably, a tale of suffering and redemption.

Drunk-driving one night, Merrick runs his car off the road and is taken in by an artisan stonecutter. On waking the next day, he finds out that the stonecutter is an acolyte of Wayne Phillips. He explains to Merrick what Phillips taught him – that every individual needs to fulfil their destiny by connecting to 'the source of infinite power.' This is implied to be the Christian God, but the way to achieve the connection is through personal conduct rather than worship (the author of the source novel was a Lutheran pastor). The would-be convert must do good without expectation of recompense of any kind – indeed they must impress upon the recipient of their kind acts the need to keep said acts secret. This is relatively easy for Merrick, who is wealthy enough to give money away, and so can ameliorate people's lot simply by reaching for his chequebook. However, when he is still dabbling with this lifestyle change, and utilising it in order to further his romantic pursuit of Helen Phillips, things go awry. During uneasy negotiations to get her to let him drive her home from a café, she steps out of his car and is hit by a passing vehicle. She survives, but has been blinded. Merrick is now truly repentant (even though, as in the case of Dr Phillips' death, no direct blame attaches to him). He makes a habit of being nearby as the now sightless Helen takes her daily constitutional; and he develops, by chance rather than design, an increasingly intimate, platonic relationship with her (he invents a pseudonym and adjusts his speaking voice slightly). Boosted by this, he sets about securing Helen's financial security by (secretive) collaborations with her lawyer, as well as persuading some of the leading neurologists in Europe to take on her case. He changes his own life, too, resuming the medical studies that he had relinquished in his misspent years. There is a watershed in the film when Helen goes to the experts in Europe in pursuit of a cure, only for them to confirm that her condition is inoperable (and therefore permanent). Merrick has followed her, and so is on hand to provide emotional support. This occasions mutual declarations of love, and the revelation, long secretly suspected by Helen, of Merrick's true identity. At the end of a perfect night on the town together, he proposes marriage and she says that she will let him know in the morning. However, when he returns the next day, he finds that she has fled with her nurse, due to fear of being a burden to him. Despite extensive searches, Merrick is unable to locate her; and is left alone to graduate and work as a dedicated surgeon in a city (i.e. municipal) hospital. (On occasion, he supplements the medical care that he provides for his patients with financial support, always on the understanding that his actions should remain secret.[58]) After several years he is contacted by the stonecutter with news that Helen is in a small town in New Mexico, in a coma and close to death. Merrick hurries to her side and discovers that her only chance of survival rests on having an operation, and that he is the only man qualified to perform it. After a momentary crisis of confidence, he operates – and as a result, both saves her life and restores her sight. The couple are reunited happily as the film ends.

It is easy to see why the high-culture police who were mentioned at the start of this chapter would scoff at the implausibility of a story like this. However, many people's lives contain unbelievable truths. Ironically, maybe, lead actress Jane Wyman had plenty of the stuff of melodrama in her own life. Adopted as a young child when her father died, she became Ronald Reagan's wife; and won her only Oscar in the year when her marriage to him broke up (which was the year after the birth and death of their third

---

58 Merrick's magnificent obsession is not so different in ethos and practice to something Hippocrates could recognise.

child).[59] Meanwhile her co-star lived most of his life under false pretences, at least in public – he was Rock Hudson, whose homosexuality only became common knowledge when he was one of the first high-profile showbiz names to die from AIDS, in 1985.

Magnificent Obsession (Stahl, 1935)

It may seem hard to credit that a film which includes all of the same story elements as the above could be classed as restrained. However, the earlier (1935) version of the movie is exactly that – on the strict understanding that we are using the term relatively.

Certainly there is little to separate the two versions in terms of the surface narrative in all its over-the-top glory.[60] The story is the same in all of its overarching aspects, and indeed some of the dialogue is repeated verbatim. (Oddly, both films were edited by the same man, too.) Interestingly, the opening scenes build up a picture of female solidarity laced with Freudian overtones. Helen – here with the surname Hudson – is portrayed as practically a sister of her husband's (i.e. Dr Hudson's) daughter Joyce, who herself is engaged to an older man. It is revealed that Helen lost her family in early childhood. There are countless two-shots of the women, emphasising their intimate relationship (as already noted, women's pictures are *about* women); and as in the later film, the husband/father–doctor is not seen (alive or dead). However, these potentially rich themes are not really followed through, the film preferring to hitch its wagon to romance. To this end, Merrick is more sympathetic throughout, and his 'good' side is revealed earlier. This downscales the 'conversion' that he undergoes; and, in direct proportion, the purgative element in the film.

In terms of stars, too, the typology is similar. Where in the later film there was Rock Hudson, here we have Robert Taylor, a leading man of the 1930s and beyond who had the enviable sobriquet of 'The Man with the Perfect Profile'; and he is paired with Irene Dunne, a well-established actress. However, by all accounts both stars had less turbulent personal lives than their successors in the roles.

---

59 She won the Oscar for her performance as a deaf-mute in a film called *Johnny Belinda* (Negulesco, 1948); and received a nomination for her role as the blinded Helen Phillips. She seems to have had a knack for playing people with sensory difficulties.

60 Indeed, in one instance, the earlier film outdoes the later one. The penitent male lead not only becomes a doctor, but he also wins a Nobel Prize for his pioneering work in brain surgery!

The bigger differences start to appear in other aspects of the film, most notably the cinematography and the music. Notwithstanding the fact that one of the background musical themes in the early film (written by famous Hollywood composer Franz Waxman) has been much borrowed since for the purpose of lampooning weepie movie scenes, music plays a much smaller role than in the later film. In the 1954 version, it is virtually a member of the cast. Furthermore, the 1935 film is in black and white; while colour is a vital part of the later version, a virtual QED of the old promotional claim 'in glorious Technicolor!'

However, let us compare two treatments of the same events, namely the episode in which Helen visits the crème de la crème of European doctors (a meeting engineered by Merrick), who after due deliberation inform her that they can be of no help to her.

The 1935 scene begins with a close-up of the plaque on the wall of the 'Institute Oculiste de Paris', almost like an intertitle in a silent movie. The 1954 version does something similar, but only after a brief scene showing Merrick at home reading a postcard from Helen explaining that tests will start the next day. Both versions then cut to a blacked-out room where the eminent doctors are examining Helen; and both make play of the contrast between light and dark, pointing up Helen's condition. In the 1935 version, the camera pans with the men as they walk across the room to confer with other colleagues, leaving Helen in her chair. There is a cutaway to Helen, sitting impassively, overhearing snatches of their cogitations. The point is thus powerfully made that they are a group, and she is on her own, with her fate out of her own hands. Two doctors come back to her and stand on either side of her as they break the bad news, one with his hand on her shoulder. As she realises that her hopes are dashed, she stands up so that she is now at their level – a self-assertive move at a moment when she might have been crushed by her circumstances. The camera dollies in to her head and shoulders, the two men being 'pushed out' from the edge of the frame. The scene lasts for just under two minutes.

There are several divergences in Sirk's approach. The first two examples relate to filming and performance, and the third to narrative structure and length. During the examination there is an extraordinary shot of a narrow torch beam being shone into Helen's eye. Surrounded by almost total darkness and occupying a small space in the centre of the screen, the light hits only the iris (not even the rest of the eyeball), creating an effect reminiscent of Samuel Beckett's celebrated close-up mouth-only play *Not I* (written over

15 years later). Whereas Beckett is thought of as 'avant-garde' and 'challenging', this shot is part of a couldn't-be-more-mainstream Hollywood movie. Wyman plays the scene differently to Dunne, too. Her face conveys the underlying worry that things are not going well, while her words are determinedly optimistic – and one of the film's recurrent motifs is the difference between appearance (e.g. of a well-heeled lifestyle) and reality (internal emotional turmoil).

The structural difference is that Sirk splits the scene in two, separating the diagnostic procedures from the moment when bad news is broken. Between them, he inserts a scene of Helen back in her hotel room, getting Joyce to write another bulletin to Merrick; who is then seen reading this and discussing it with a senior colleague at his hospital. The main effect of this material, as with the previous postcard-reading scene, is to integrate Merrick (and his romance with Helen) more thoroughly into the story.[61] However, it also serves to prolong and heighten the build-up to Helen's fall in the second medical scene (tying in with her verbal rationalisations). In this, the doctors are as solicitous and kindly, and at first surround (and thus envelop) her, as before ('before' meaning both the earlier scene and the earlier film); but soon Helen's irreducible isolation is accentuated by the blocking of the actors and the arrangement of the scenery (effectively bisecting the frame at one point), not to mention the replacement of pans and medium shots that accommodate all of the characters by a shot–countershot strategy that individualises. (In general, Stahl likes longer takes, whereas Sirk favours more frequent cuts that serve to heat up the proceedings.) We could also consider Helen's outfit (it is hardly an exaggeration to say that the state of Sirk's heroines can be accurately gauged by their clothing); and some clever business with the track blinds in the doctor's office (almost every interior scene in the film has an exterior included in it somewhere); and a few other things besides (e.g. the second consultation scene lasts three minutes, so is nearly half as long again as in the 1935 film, and that does not include the diagnostic scene).

---

61 This point is further emphasised by the stupendous dissolve that joins the two scenes. Merrick is on the left of the frame, facing the so-called fourth wall (i.e. the cinema auditorium). Helen comes into the frame from the right and turns to go in through the door to the Institute. As the images overlap, she appears to be walking towards him just as he is thinking of her. To top this off, the Institute has a glass frontage that is reflecting the leafy urban undulations. As Helen walks in through the door it seems as if she is being absorbed by her environment – that is to say, her identity is being subsumed by her situation.

At any rate, I hope it is clear that where Stahl opts for an elegant, understated directorial style, Sirk prefers to fire on all cylinders (although this is not to be mistaken for a lack of sophistication). There is little subtext to the 1935 film – the audience is invited to feel the emotions of Merrick and Hudson, to stay on the bucking bronco of the storyline, and to gain pleasure from that process. It is a moral tale, to be sure, but a relatively straightforward one notwithstanding. Sirk does that job, too, and he has to, arguably, if he is not to lose his audience. However, he also conveys other things at the same time; and manages to insinuate them into the film in such a way that they might not be noticed (primarily achieving them by visual rather than narrative means). For instance, the sets and props suggest that he is commenting on American society in the Eisenhower years, showing the era's almost fetishistic materialism and its shadow – an underlying existential anxiety.

Considerations

It is a pity that space precludes substantial discussion of other excellent medically tinged melodramas such as *Kings Row* (1942, Wood) and *Suddenly Last Summer* (1956, Mankiewicz). There is a plurality in their representations of doctors that is very interesting; and the former can be seen chronologically (in the context of this chapter) as a bridge between the two versions of *Magnificent Obsession*, since the story of individuals' tribulations is played out in a specific social setting (a generic American small town in the early part of the twentieth century).

However, the brace of *Magnificent Obsessions* raise enough important issues on their own. First, we can note that doctors in melodramas often seem to occupy the calm space, their role being to help others to cope with catastrophe by deploying rational thought and deed. Thus they are bastions of logical positivism, even (or perhaps especially!) when they are contending with emotionally charged issues. Medicine repairs physical damage (in this case, blindness), and in so doing restores social (not to say sexual) order (the widow Helen is re-partnered; and the selfish womaniser Merrick signs up to monogamy and social responsibility).

The second point is more general, and moot. By blasting their way out of the confines of good taste and restraint, melodramas can reach parts that other films do not.[62] For instance, they can address issues that are usually

---

62 Although they are less popular in mainstream US cinema than they used to be, some of their sexual and social themes have been appropriated by television soaps (from

repressed because they are messy or untoward. This culture of excess can beget two audience responses which, although opposite, may not be mutually exclusive. The first is alienation (or what is sometimes called 'distanciation') – the 'high-culture' position, we could say, where the spectator observes proceedings uninterestedly (if not with a hint of disdain). The second is the inverse, namely identification, with its good companion vicariousness. Here the spectator becomes involved with the characters and their life events, and so is transported emotionally. Curiously, people can find themselves experiencing both reactions during the same film – think of the not infrequently heard remark, 'The movie was a load of rubbish, but I cried at the end!,' a description of someone being ambushed by ambivalence. In this case, the ambivalence hinges on the paradoxical coexistence of empathy and detachment – two words that one hears a lot when doctor–patient relationships are being discussed. Doctors have to confront bodies (and accompanying psyches) that are abnormal, sometimes *in extremis* – bones that are smashed, hearts that are attacked, cells that are multiplying uncontrollably, agitated mental states that are uncontained – conditions that might be described as biologically melodramatic. Maybe a melodramatic plot descending on a hapless character (i.e. external agencies or events having a violent impact on an individual's life) is akin to someone falling sick, disease having invaded their body and jolted their biosystems. At any rate, doctors' response to all of this, most sages agree, has to be a nicely judged mixture of scientific detachment and emotional empathy. There appear, then, to be parallels between the doctor–patient relationship and the spectator–film relationship. Plainly, doctors intervene in events, whereas spectators do not; but before, during and after those interventions, a doctor is responding consciously and unconsciously, emotionally and intellectually, to the story in front of him or her, just like a moviegoer.

Perhaps medical school curricula should include a compulsory course on melodrama . . .

References

Finler JW. *The Movie Directors Story*. London: Octopus Books; 1985.

Further reading

Gibbs J. *Mise-en-scene: film style and interpretation*. London: Wallflower Press; 2003.
Various. *Book of the Cinema*. London: Mitchell Beazley; 1979.

Peyton Place to *Desperate Housewives* via *Dallas*) and arthouse directors (think David Lynch or Pedro Almodovar or Todd Haynes).

Filmography

MAGNIFICENT OBSESSION (1935)

Credits

Director	John M Stahl
Producers	Carl Laemmle, John M Stahl
Production Company	Universal
Screenplay	Sarah Mason, Victor Heerman, George O'Neill
Original story	Lloyd C Douglas
Photography	John Mescall
Editor	Milton Carruth
Art Director	Charles Hall
Music	Franz Waxman

Cast

Robert Merrick	Robert Taylor
Helen Hudson	Irene Dunne
Joyce Hudson	Betty Furness
Nancy Johnson	Sara Haden
Edward Randolph	Ralph Morgan

MAGNIFICENT OBSESSION (1954)

Credits

Director	Douglas Sirk
Producer	Ross Hunter
Production Company	Universal
Screenplay	Robert Blees, Wells Root
Original story	Lloyd C Douglas
Photography	Russell Metty
Editor	Milton Carruth
Art Director	Bernard Herzbrun, Emrich Nicholson
Set Director	Russell Gausman, Ruby Levitt
Music	Frank Skinner

Cast

Bob Merrick	Rock Hudson
Helen Phillips	Jane Wyman
Joyce Phillips	Barbara Rush
Nancy Ashford	Agnes Moorehead
Edward Randolph	Otto Kruger

CHAPTER 14

Mirror, mirror, on the screen

In films, a hospital can be just a hospital (i.e. the physical and social setting in which a particular medical or other story happens, as for example in movies like *Awakenings*, which was discussed in Chapter 9); or it can be a more symbolic space, a forum for the debate about the health or otherwise of the body politic – a place where some of society's current concerns manifest themselves.[63] The divide is not absolute, and overlaps occur in several films that have already been discussed in this book (e.g. *The Doctor*, and others in Chapter 12). Nonetheless, the films that are considered in this chapter all take place in hospital settings and – if we presume to guess at their main underlying purpose – are fairly and squarely designed to hold a mirror up to a wider social context. The angle at which that mirror is held, and its size and shape, vary of course.

The Hospital (Hiller, 1971)

The film announces itself with a pre-title voice-over sequence chronicling an instance of iatrogenesis that would have had Ivan Illich (the Austrian philosopher, rather than Tolstoy's similarly named fictional invalid) making copious notes. An accumulation of heedlessness, selfish behaviour and straightforward incompetence on the part of health professionals causes a man's death late at night in the bowels of a large New York Hospital. The film's central character, Dr Herb Bock, summarises the events trenchantly: 'The entire machinery of modern medicine has apparently conspired to kill one lousy patient!'

---

63 Both approaches provide social comment – the former indirectly and perhaps unwittingly, and the latter directly and definitely wittingly.

Bock is the film's hook – the protagonist whose story carries the themes of the film at the same time as giving us access to other characters' stories. Played by George C Scott with his dial set at maximum ferocity, he embodies one form of the American Dream. The only child of poor immigrant parents, his intellectual aptitude has enabled him to rocket to success in the respected and worthy field of medical practice (a 'boy genius' who becomes 'my son the doctor'). He passionately believes in the profession of medicine, citing it as the greatest love of his life, his vehicle for achieving 'a sense of permanent worth'; and he believes that as 'chief of medicine at one of the great hospitals, I am a necessary person.' He even takes his junior doctor teaching responsibilities seriously!

Despite this, or in part because of it, he finds himself in the midst of a middle-age middle-class menopausal meltdown ('I'm 53 years old, with all the attendant fears', he tells a solicitous colleague). His marriage has collapsed, he is estranged from his rebellious children, and he is impotent – both sexually, which he doesn't mind too much, and in terms of his desire to work, about which he does mind. Suicide is a distinct possibility.

However, all of this personal stuff dovetails with a world around him that is also falling apart. At one point Bock says 'We have established the most enormous medical identity ever conceived and people are sicker than ever. We cure nothing. We heal nothing. . . . Half the kids in the ghetto out there haven't even been inoculated for polio.' When a junior nurse reports to the nurses' station that there is an unidentified dead man in bed 806, the sister expresses neither surprise nor concern, nor does she (for what seems like an age) even get up to investigate further. She merely replies 'I don't know what you're talking about', a mantra that she repeats in a monotone several times as the nurse tries to rouse her to action by restating the facts. This is a world in which basic human responses have been replaced by a mentality of banal bureaucracy. Another scene shows a harassed administrator, who is trying to keep tabs on comings and goings in the casualty department, shouting at an unresponsive patient that he will not be permitted to leave until she has his insurance details – not noticing that he is dead. (As may be gleaned, the film is often humorous, but not in such a way that you find yourself laughing.) The hospital is besieged by angry community groups objecting to its scheme to build a new wing on land that has been marked for slum clearance. The chief executive runs the gauntlet of their ire each day as he arrives at work; and at one point near the end of the film, during a particularly confrontational meeting with the protesters, he quits his job on the spot and hands over the reins of power ('Fine – *you* take over. *You* fight the government. *You* fight the unions. *You* fight the lawsuits. *You* try to keep on budget.'). Later, a riot breaks out involving the same malcontents. 'The whole wounded madhouse of our times' is how one patient describes things – a phrase that captures the despairing liberal sensibility underlying the film. Certainly, if the sickness lies in society, then it is not curable by doctors (notwithstanding the fact that some of them are part of the problem).

So society is portrayed as being in an advanced state of collapse, and the film's sympathies lie with Bock and his kind (i.e. white, middle-aged men) rather than, for instance, with the multi-ethnic protesting youths from the local community. (The film is written, produced and directed by such men, too.) In the event, the movie's ending turns out to be mildly upbeat. Bock doesn't run away (either by killing himself or by eloping with his new young love interest), but opts instead to stay and carry on the fight. 'I can't walk out when the hospital is falling apart. Someone has to be responsible' (this as he and the chief executive walk back into the fray at the hospital's main entrance). Post-war liberalism has had a near-death experience and survived.[64]

Britannia Hospital (Anderson, 1982)

It is said that England is always 10 years behind the USA, so *Britannia Hospital* is dated about right. The 'message' of the film is fairly clear from the title. This is full-blown allegory – the state of the nation as revealed by goings on at one of its hospitals. A transatlantic transposition, then, of *The Hospital*? Yes, and in spades (the film even starts with a similar unnoticed and unloved patient's death).[65] Whereas *The Hospital* took place near the out-

---

64 Genealogists of American film might trace a line from *The Hospital* through to *Critical Care* (Lumet, 1997) via movies such as *Where Does It Hurt?* (Amateau, 1972), *House Calls* (Zieff, 1974) and *Critical Condition* (Apted, 1987) – a social-comment-cum-comedy collection.

65 However, outside the context of this chapter it would be dangerous to try to tie this kind of sequential bow too tightly. *Britannia Hospital* was made by English director Lindsay Anderson, an inveterate lancer of social boils, whose anger at the attendant pus was established long before this film. Far from being a quick-fire response to topical social turmoil, *Britannia Hospital* is in fact the final instalment in a loose trilogy of films that Anderson began in 1968 with *If. . .*, a startling, semi-fantastical anti-Establishment tale set in a public school. In between came *O Lucky Man!* (1975) (another condemnation of British mores), the link between the three films being the character played by Malcolm McDowell (called Mick Travis, although in truth his name provides pretty much the only continuity between the roles).

skirts of a conurbation called Believable, its exaggeration and outcry rooted in a realistic tradition, *Britannia Hospital* is situated well outside that city's limits. A commentator, speaking about another of the director's films,[66] sums this up nicely: '[The film deals in] reality, not realism. It's about the nervous breakdown of English society.' Exit a central protagonist around whom the story strands (and sympathies) coalesce, to be replaced by a series of diverse sub-plots; enter extra social sideswipes, with the monarchy, religion and the media coming in for scathing treatment, along with 'traditional' targets such as healthcare staff self-interest, endemic social inefficiency and substandard industrial (i.e. hospital) systems and facilities. The notional plot driver is a planned royal visit to Britannia Hospital. The imminence of this event turns up the heat under various simmering pots, including works department staff who are working to rule during problematic negotiations with management ('An insult to me is an insult to every non-skilled operative in this hospital!'); catering staff who threaten to down utensils because the royal lunch is being supplied by Fortnum & Mason rather than being cooked on the premises; other hospital staff who are on strike because of the presence in the private patients' wing of a foreign military dictator; tension concerning the general provision of private patients' services (not to mention the increasingly vocal dissatisfaction of the private patients themselves); rivalrous consultants; and so on. The wily and indefatigable head administrator attempts to keep the peace initially by hook, but eventually by crook, his increasingly desperate actions depriving the audience of the only character in whom they had any kind of rooting interest.

In fact, the film has very little to do with medicine *per se* (apart from one Frankenstein-type storyline). It is more interested in assembling a national social mosaic, where the background (bomb attacks in central London, road accidents, transport strikes, TV technicians' degeneracy) is as important as the central action. Yet a hospital was surely not an arbitrary choice of setting; on the contrary, it is a near-perfect one, providing a place where an infinitely broad cross-section of people and social groups can plausibly appear and interact. Moreover, the film's location provides an extra layer (or two) of irony. Most of the external scenes and some of the interiors were shot at Friern Hospital in North London. This was formerly called Colney Hatch Lunatic Asylum, one of the original and largest Victorian mental asylums (the name

---

66 Musician Alan Price, talking about *O Lucky Man!* in the DVD version's special features section.

'Colney Hatch' at one time being slang for 'madhouse') – a fact that must have greatly appealed to the film-makers! However, what they would not have known was that, a decade or so after the film was made, the hospital and much of its extensive surrounding land would be sold under the directions of the contemporary Conservative government to property developers – as unequivocal and symbolic a sign of the times as any that Anderson had dreamt up!

Syndromes and a Century (2006, Weerasethakul)

Jumping from the previous two films into this one is like swimming underwater in the Pacific Ocean after cycling up the Rockies (or Mount Snowdon) – you're on the same planet, but almost every other sensation is different. Certainly *Syndromes and a Century* (made by a Thai director with international financing) works its wonders in mysterious ways; and patience might be a necessary virtue for viewers who are unaccustomed to its particular modus operandi. It is set in contemporary Thailand, mostly in two healthcare institutions (a futuristic hospital and a less modern local clinic); and the majority of the central protagonists are healthcare staff and patients. So far, so similar to our two preceding films; but things take a different turn thereafter.

In place of what one critic called the 'speechifying' of *The Hospital*, wherein people are constantly making pronouncements that seem to be aimed at the audience as much as to the other characters, the dialogue in *Syndromes and a Century* proceeds almost as if the cinema auditorium does not exist. (That is to say, we feel like witnesses to it, rather than collateral targets.) Where Dr Bock might harangue us with a diatribe about the youth of today in a sharp-as-a-tack, eminently quotable monologue, the central female doctor in *Syndromes and a Century* is liable to ask a job applicant, quite non-sequentially, what DDT stands for – a question whose significance only becomes slightly clearer about 90 minutes further into the film.

The same is true with regard to plot. There is almost nothing in the way of storyline to push the film forward (in contrast to the competing sub-plots of *Britannia Hospital*, which are all on an inexorable forward march). Even when we think that we have alighted on one (an unfolding love affair, for instance), it tends to melt back into the bushes before it reaches any kind of resolution. From the beginning to the end, notwithstanding some subtle changes along the way, the storytelling style in *Syndromes and a Century* can be said to be the opposite of a tirade, preferring an allusive (even elusive) approach. There is more showing than telling; and what is being shown is not necessarily a story *per se*. This is a welcome variation in a world (and not just a cinematic world) that is usually enamoured of narratives. Here conventional narrative is given a thorough going over – stories are started (or are joined somewhere in the middle) and never finished (even those that are told in flashback); or they get repeated with different protagonists in different places. Closure was evidently a word that was banned from the set. All of this might leave the viewer pondering what exactly the film *does* concern itself with. This is a question that is best answered by people watching the film for themselves. However, to this writer, some of the things the film is *about* include the following:[67]

➤ what might be described as 'cultural shoulder-rubbing' – in contrast to the polarisation and confrontation favoured by most mainstream cinema. For instance, we see an outpatient clinic consultation in which the patient, a Buddhist monk, and the young female doctor have a dialogue that reveals their different belief systems. Sometimes their explanatory models conflict, sometimes they concur (or at least overlap), and at one intoxicating moment there is a commingling of Freud, physiology and karma in the air! No one's dogma prevails

➤ male–female relationships – there are several romances at different stages of development (they are often unrequited, as one might expect from a film that rejects narrative templates); and there is an intriguing (non-gay) male–male relationship, too

➤ communalism – people agglomerate throughout the film, under various unifying banners that range from uniforms to group activities

➤ the relationship between nature and man, as shown particularly by the interface between buildings (both old and new) and vegetation. There are countless inside-out shots (for instance, an office with a verdant exterior visible through a window). The film was banned in Thailand (a possible badge of honour?), and one assumes that this was because it contains 'subversive' images of a monk playing a guitar, semi-alcoholic doctors drinking during work time (and on work premises), and hospital scenes featuring casualties of the Thai regime's social and military policies. The latter tend to appear in the second half of the film, and it is noticeable that the implied harmony of the shots (in the first half) that

---

67 Really no film should be laid out in bullet points – such an approach is too reminiscent of a corpse on a mortuary slab; but this one is surely opaque enough to resist the most reductive typography.

contain man-made objects (buildings) and nature is replaced by the angst that emanates from scenes in windowless basements.

Not only is this film is almost entirely plotless, but also it is filmed and soundtracked unusually. One striking feature is the overwhelming preponderance of long takes filmed by a fixed camera.[68] Regardless of the action (or lack of it) that is being filmed, this shooting style makes the movie feel 'slow.' The carefully controlled use of colours also tends to lend an air of artificiality, although there is nothing fantastical in what is shown; while the background music, when it is deployed, consists largely of sustained polychromatic chords (almost like a dirge) rather than melodies, and seems designed to unsettle. (Compare this with the cinematographic strategies of films such as *The Hospital* or *Britannia Hospital* and you could almost be talking about two different art forms. Yet all of these films are undoubtedly critiques of the condition of the societies in which they are situated.)

Does all of this make the film hard to understand? Only insofar as it deviates from the norm of most films that most people see, and therefore offers a somewhat unfamiliar experience. Here one should recall FD Roosevelt's line about having nothing to fear but fear itself, and guard against the habitual desire to ascribe simple cause-and-effect-type explanations to everything that happens on a cinema screen. Poetic contemplation is a less common mode of address than information-laden didacticism in the cinema (as in life), but is no less valid.

This chapter could have headed off in several other directions. For instance, it would be quite possible to consider a separate group of films that see institutions as vehicles for social control or even repression. The fascistic mental hospital in *One Flew Over The Cuckoo's Nest* (Foreman, 1972) is perhaps the *ne plus ultra* of a group that might also include *Suddenly Last Summer* (Mankiewicz, 1956) and even – a good way back down the continuum – *Doctor In The House* (Thomas, 1954). Or one might have looked at films that use the hospital as a test-tube for social mixing – for instance, Ingmar Bergman's *So Close To Life* (1958) or *The National Health* (Gold, 1979). In these films, patients with diverse social and psychological backgrounds

---

68 When the approach is altered, the effect is striking. At one point a character (followed by a suddenly very mobile camera) goes on a long, circuitous journey down into the depths of the hospital to the section reserved for military patients. This is surely conveying how Thailand's military troubles have been suppressed, denied and buried.

are thrown together and the audience gets to watch the sparks that fly. And so on – the artistic potential that a healthcare setting has to offer is almost limitless.

Further reading

Milne T. *Monthly Film Bulletin* 1972; **39**: 95–6.
Stuart A. *Films and Filming* 1972; **18**: 50.

Filmography

THE HOSPITAL (1971)

Credits

Director	Arthur Hiller
Producer	Howard Gottfried
Production Company	United Artists
Screenplay	Paddy Chayefsky
Photography	Victor Kemper
Editor	Eric Albertson
Production Design	Gene Rudolph
Music	Morris Surdin

Cast

Dr Herb Bock	George C Scott
Barbara Drummond	Diana Rigg
Edmund Drummond	Barnard Hughes
Dr Welbeck	Richard Dysart

BRITANNIA HOSPITAL (1982)

Credits

Director	Lindsay Anderson
Producers	Davina Belling, Clive Parsons
Production Company	Film and General Productions
Screenplay	David Sherwin
Photography	Mike Fash
Editor	Michael Ellis
Production Design	Norris Spencer
Music	Alan Price

Cast

Vincent Potter	Leonard Rossiter
Matron	Vivian Pickles
Professor Millar	Graham Crowden

Sir Geoffrey Brockenhurst	Peter Jeffrey
Nurse Amanda Persil	Marsha Hunt
Ben Keating	Robin Askwith
Mick Travis	Malcolm McDowell
Red	Mark Hamill
Sir Anthony Mount	Marcus Powell

SYNDROMES AND A CENTURY (2006)

Credits

Director	Apichatpong Weerasethakul
Producers	Simon Field, Pantham Thongsangl
Production Company	New Crowned Hope, Thai Independent Filmmakers Alliance, Kick The Machine
Screenplay	Apichatpong Weerasethakul
Photography	Sayombhu Mukdeeprom
Editor	Lee Chatametikool
Art Director	Akekarat Homlaor
Music	Kantee Anantagant

Cast

Dr Wan	Wanna Wattanajinda
Dr Tei	Nantarat Sawaddikul
Pa Jane	Jenjira Pongpas
Old monk	Sin Kaewpakpin
Ple	Arkanae Cherkam
Dr Nohng	Jaruchai Iamaram

CHAPTER 15

In closing

The end of the book is nigh, a circumstance that makes the author more aware than ever of what is *not* in these pages. (You will gather that this is a pre-emptive attempt to repent my sins of commission – those of omission will no doubt be brought to my attention in due course!)

For instance, there could have been chapters on medical thrillers, such as *Coma* (Crichton, 1976), its ancestor *Green for Danger* (Gilliat, 1946) and its descendant *Extreme Measures* (Apted, 1996) (not to mention *The Fugitive* (Davis, 1993) or *Tell No One* (Canet, 2006); or medical comedies (from silent movies featuring Fatty Arbuckle and Buster Keaton to more recent successes such as *Analyse This* (Ramis, 1999) via the Marx Brothers' *A Day At The Races* (Wood, 1937).[69] And what about documentaries? What about films that focus on public health issues, or in which doctors are embedded in specific communities? And so on – the possibilities are virtually inexhaustible, and consequently so are the grounds for accusations of oversight.

Yet there are particular films that it is especially regrettable have not found their way into this book. Examples in random order include *Sunday, Bloody Sunday* (Schlesinger, 1971); *The Lost One* (Lorre, 1951); *The English Surgeon* (Smith, 2008); *The Citadel* (Vidor, 1938); *Not As A Stranger* (Kramer, 1955); *The Doctor's Dilemma* (Asquith, 1958); *A Man To Remember* (Kanin, 1938); *Send Me No Flowers* (Jewison, 1964); *Dead Ringers* (Cronenberg, 1988) and two films by Edmund Goulding, *We Are Not Alone* (1939) and *Nightmare Alley* (1947); not to mention the important trio of films that featured Sidney

---

69 A good chapter has already been written by Graeme Harper on one tranche of these (Harper G. 'Either he's dead or my watch has stopped': medical notes in 1930s film comedy. In: Harper G, Moor A (eds) *Signs of Life: medicine and cinema*, London: Wallflower Press; 2005.)

Poitier as a doctor,[70] offering three different takes on racism; and *The Death Of Mr Lazarescu* (Puiu, 2005). Some of the above are just very interesting doctor films; others are outstanding works of art in their own right, and will repay many times over whatever time and trouble are required to locate and watch them. My only extenuation for their absence is that they are too rich and complex not to have a whole chapter devoted to each, and that so much additional material would have made this volume unwieldy.

At any rate, this incompleteness is supporting evidence for my belief that the subject of doctors in the movies is a fantastically rich one that has been relatively underexplored. It is a broad and deep territory, and much of it remains uncharted, both descriptively and with regard to theoretical concerns. I therefore very much hope that this book will stimulate further enquiry of an academic nature; and that it will also persuade readers to draw up their own film-watching menu purely for personal pleasure.

---

70 *No Way Out* (Mankiewicz, 1950), *Pressure Point* (Cornfield, 1962) and *Guess Who's Coming To Dinner* (Kramer, 1967).

General bibliography

Alexander M, Lenahan P, Pavlov A. *Cinemeducation: a comprehensive guide to using film in medical education*. Oxford: Radcliffe Publishing; 2005.

Bordwell D. *Narration in the Fiction Film*. London: Routledge; 1987.

Bordwell D, Thompson K. *Film Art*. New York: McGraw-Hill Education; 2000.

Cartwright L. *Screening the Body*. Minneapolis, MN: University of Minnesota Press; 1995.

Conrad P. *To Be Continued: four stories and their survival*. Oxford: Clarendon Press; 1995.

Dans P. *Doctors in the Movies*. Bloomington, IL: Medi-Ed Press; 2000.

Elena A. Exemplary lives: biographies of scientists on the screen. *Public Underst Sci.* 1993; **2**: 205–23.

Elena A. Skirts in the lab: 'Madame Curie' and the image of the woman scientist in the feature film. *Public Underst Sci.* 1997; **6**: 269–78.

Flores G. Doctors in the movies: healers, heels, and Hollywood. *Arch Dis Child.* 2004; **89**: 1084–8.

Frayling C. *Mad, Bad and Dangerous: the scientist and the cinema*. London: Reaktion Books; 2005.

Friedman LD (ed.) *Cultural Sutures: medicine and media*. Durham, NC: Duke University Press; 2004.

Gabbard GO (ed.) *Psychoanalysis and Film*. London: Karnac; 2001.

Gianetti L. *Understanding Movies*. Upper Saddle River, NJ: Prentice Hall; 1996.

Harper G, Moor A (eds) *Signs of Life: medicine and cinema*. London: Wallflower Press; 2005.

Hayward S. *Key Concepts in Cinema Studies*. London: Routledge; 1999.

Helman C. *The Body of Frankenstein's Monster*. London: WW Norton Company; 1992.

Henderson B. Two types of film theory. *Film Quart.* 1971; **24**: 33–42.

Heyward Brock D. The doctor as dramatic hero. *Perspect Biol Med.* 1991; **34**: 279–95.

Jouhanneau J. Les scientifiques vus par les cineastes. In: Martinet A (ed.) *Le Cinéma et la Science*. Paris: CNRS Éditions; 1994. pp. 248–61.

Moody N, Hallam J (eds) *Medical Fictions*. Liverpool: Liverpool John Moores University Press; 1998.

Paietta A, Kauppila J. *Health Professionals on Screen*. London: Scarecrow Press; 1999.

Rosenstone RA. Comments on science in the visual media. *Public Underst Sci*. 2003; **12**: 335–9.

Rosenstone RA. *History on Film/Film on History*. Harlow: Pearson Education; 2006.

Shortland M. Screen memories: towards a history of psychiatry and psychoanalysis in the movies. *Br J Hist Sci*. 1987; **20**: 421–52.

Shortland M. *Medicine and Film: a checklist, survey and research resource*. Oxford: Wellcome Unit for the History of Medicine; 1989.

Turner G. *Film as Social Practice*. London: Routledge; 1993.

Wood A. *Technoscience in Contemporary Film*. Manchester: Manchester University Press; 2002.

Index

T - #0673 - 101024 - C0 - 246/174/9 - PB - 9781846191572 - Gloss Lamination